HEALING THROUGH
COLOUR

HEALING THROUGH COLOUR

THEO GIMBEL

SAFFRON WALDEN
THE C. W. DANIEL COMPANY LIMITED

First published in Great Britain
by the C. W. Daniel Company Limited
1 Church Path, Saffron Walden,
Essex, CB10 1JP, England

SBN 85207 156 6
Reprinted 1983, 1985

Printed and bound in Great Britain
by The Burlington Press (Cambridge) Ltd,
Station Road, Foxton, Cambridge CB2 6SW

Contents

Preface

This work started some twenty-five years ago when I became a teacher at St Christopher's School in Bristol. The children at this school are all in need of healing and the teachers have to be therapists, going beyond the normal bounds of teaching. I started there in 1950, and much of my knowledge has been acquired under the loving influence of Catherine Grace, the founder of that school. About halfway through my time there I found myself involved in research into colour and light and their application to art.

I grew up in close contact with the teaching of Rudolf Steiner and still treasure the memory of meeting him when I was a small boy. One of the main things that I learnt from this early time at Dornach was how the work of all the spiritual teachers blends together. Hence the studios I now run, Hygeia, are places where the masters of all the ages can meet without conflict, each adding another aspect to the whole of man and his part in this world's evolution. Through the right techniques, which we must employ in the work of healing, we can be assured of the right communication with the spiritual worlds.

Thus I see that Rudolf Steiner brings the spiritual thinking, Pierre Teilhard de Chardin adds the spiritual action of will, and my friend Andrew Glazewski the universal love; while Carl Jung opens the soul of man and looks deeply into the images which feature in the visions of each individual. In direct reference to this I must express my eternal gratitude to Bruce Macmanaway, the finest and most efficient disciplinarian in spiritual work. Without his guidance I would not allow myself to embark upon such work.

It is with love and gratitude that I acknowledge these masters, but one more must be given his rightful place as the foundationstone of this work, which is done in the name of Hygeia, the great Goddess of Healing – and that is the master of all, Pythagoras.

A book of this kind not only touches on the vast subject of colour, but also on all that, in one way or another, has to be linked with it. We need to understand man if we are to heal him. To try to understand this being is a life-long undertaking. This book is not a complete, definitive work on colour therapy, but a modest start for the student who wishes to study this vast field.

I must also express my special thanks to Patricia Fountain, who not only did all the initial typing but corrected and re-phrased many of the lines which were lacking clarity.

To all the counsellors at Hygeia must go my very special gratitude, above all Sir John Langman, Bart., as it is through their support that I am able to do all the research and development work. And further thanks to the Ven. Richard Traynor for reading through the chapters one by one; to my family, who reluctantly let me disappear for much longer than usual, even on holidays, to continue this work; and to countless people who have offered help in all ways, whose names would fill a chapter at least.

Acknowledgements are due to Leslie Scolfour who took all the photographs. The drawings are all by the author.

Chapter 1

Introduction

How My Work Began

This book was not thought of, nor had I any intention at the time about investigating colour, art, light and form when, in 1961 (after the celebration of the anniversary of Rudolf Steiner's birth), I started some painting classes for adults after my school work with children at St Christopher's School was over for the day.

It was there, through John Cosh and his wife, that I met Mary Fraser, who later said: 'There are similarities between what you said about the healing art of mosaics, and the way in these early centuries after Christ the artists pieced together the broken vision which man needs to proceed on the path.' Incidentally, we have almost reached the same stage again now.

All these links, and many more, grew out of that period and many things combined to change my views on colour. Totally untrained, I started to investigate because I felt there was more to discover. I discovered more because I had no training. I could, as it were, put 2 and 1 together and still make 4 because the unthought-of and the as yet unseen often emerge from the non-professional approach. One apparently does things all wrong and occasionally there emerges a new concept.

What has been lost in the past is often rediscovered, with a new aspect, on another level of consciousness. I woke up and how it all started became very clear to me. The details may find a place in a future book which may one day be written as a sequel to the present one.

Dr Hans Jenny was our family doctor during the years

1937–49. I owe him much of my present state of good health, in particular when he collected me from the hills with a broken spine in January 1939. Through his wisdom I am, today, totally mobile. Hans Jenny had enormous ESP and could therefore decide on important matters such as when to put a broken limb into plaster or when not. With three ribs broken and two vertebrae smashed, he left me in my mother's house, lying on an ordinary bed, not in plaster, and through gentle movement during the next ten days I retained the mobility of my spine. Later, in the army, I was a unique, much-X-rayed private, whose spine was often an inexplicable miracle to surgeons.

It was this, in fact, and similar experiences which made me think later that there must be more to so-called common sense and logic than meets the eye. If there are people who can actually see more, hear more or are better able to 'perceive knowledge', through which organs do these extra-sensory perceptions find their entrance to the brain? Or do they perhaps come to the heart first and we then spend a lot of time transmitting them to our brains, often only to find that we have made a great mess and tangle out of the original perception, having lost the truth and purity of the heart's knowledge? Women are much better at preservation of the original, and they do lead us men, often unwillingly, back to the heart truth and the real wisdom.

Today I know for certain that Hans Jenny, and many others whom I have had the privilege to meet, use this capacity far more often than is apparent. Extra-sensory perceptions are often much later verified by long, patiently pursued research, when in fact they have been applied over and over again successfully. Many a man would have died if the scientific proof of his condition had had to be produced before he could be treated. Lifetimes and whole fortunes are spent on research, but often very little, if indeed anything, has a practical application. Often the field of research is so narrow that the implications of its results are lost.

The Need to Recover ESP Powers

Shelley and his contemporaries did not possess knowledge of

electronics or microscopes of present-day magnifying capacity to enable them to understand the behaviour of the atom. But consider the following passage:

> A sphere, which is as many thousand
> Solid as crystal, yet through all its
> Flow, as through empty space music and light
> Ten thousand orbs involving and involved,
> Purple and azure, white and green and golden
> ... thousand sightless axles spinning ...
>
> (P. B. Shelley, 1819)

Richard Holmes, in his work *Shelley, the Pursuit*, points out that the approach of an artistic mind, art in its creative moment, often has access to knowledge which comes to the scientist only a century or so later. Shelley is not the only one who provided us with a very clear picture of the atom or the universe long before physics discovered them. Schiller in his work is accurate in his history; yet, at the time he wrote his dramas, historical records of the lives of Mary Stuart (and Elizabeth I of England) and Don Juan were not to be found in any books. The artistic mind, it seems, has access to the world fountain of knowledge through ESP.

ESP and the old wisdom of the sacred races, whom we have been so busy stamping out of existence, may well be the only way in which to save this planet. Races such as the Mayas, Incas and, more recently, the Red Indians, maintained a close link between their whole environment and their bodies, and listened to nature. This attitude kept alive that we call now ESP – we once had it and lost it and now we must regain it on a new level of consciousness.

It is not the intention of those who are really helpers on this planet to supplant or to push out of their places those who are serving in a profession, but rather to be involved as a further aid to understanding our own task. This is done with the greatest possible humility and sense of service. Let there be no blame attached to the shortcomings of anyone. But let there be a sense of co-operation and 're-search' (meaning to re-find what has gone, lost in the past).

Relation of Colour and Sound to Medicine

The Eternal Music which originally composed the visible forms (and still does, although we do not seem to hear it any longer) is now recognised as being able to help in the medical treatment of illness. We are now realising that colour can play an equal role as we begin to understand its significance as a servant in the medical world today. Neither colour nor sound replaces any of the medical work of a doctor, but both offer a more complete treatment to medicine.

When the energies present in all living matter are considered, it can be seen that they always go in pairs. The components of each pair are in polarity opposition; each pair has a positive and a negative element. The terms male and female will be used to describe these energies. When the term female or male, positive or negative, occurs in the text, the reader may take it, not as measures of good or bad, but as one of the equal, complementary energies which there are working in man, through man, to create a third, higher energy which we cannot always see straight away, nor understand.

What is lacking today in most areas of education is an understanding that all continuity, security and sense of purpose depend on a knowledge which gives man a grasp of his origins. We need a vision that can really lead us again, yes, lead us back to paradise. Hence it will be necessary to introduce the personalities who were outstanding at the beginning of the fifth post-atlantean epoch; in other words, some 2,600 years ago. They hold the links between one age and the other, the old and the new. In particular there are the two whom we shall have to take very seriously into account: Pythagoras and Hippocrates.

A Vision for the Future

Several of our own contemporaries are at the same stage, linked to the roots. Rudolf Steiner, Blavatski, Teilhard de Chardin and Andrew Glazewski are but a few of the outstanding ones. Undoubtedly each individual human being in each age serves on many levels; none is immaterial or trivial. Physicists and scientists in medical fields are, because of many unsolved questions and a few significant insights into human nature, led to ways of thinking which help to create a vision for the future. As they work they find that the answers are not all 'in the book', but are perhaps as yet unwritten in the hearts of men and women who have access to full knowledge once they allow their thoughts to become free enough to wander along the untrodden paths of the mind. There, in a dream, is often revealed the truth; and its logical use in our daily environment takes so much love and patience to realise that it has sometimes broken even the greatest among us. To mind comes the late husband of my very special friend Dame Isobel Cripps, Sir Stafford Cripps. The truth of the old saying 'mind over matter' is often demonstrated when the intuitive mind finds solutions which are totally unexpected but absolutely right. That such discoveries via the intuitive path do work out, and that excellent results achieved, is something that those with a strictly logical approach find at times most difficult to see, let alone trust enough to try out, even if it were only to satisfy their own curiosity.

It is in moments of real crisis, when at the brink of death – as I have been several times – that we actually use, albeit in desperation, our intuitive or, say, spiritual energies; they lead us to a place where we are saved from the impending disaster and in that moment of relaxation we have no words, statistics or scientific handbook to tell us how we got out of the impossible situation. Are these things which happen almost daily, then, untrue? Do not people live now who, by the normal course of events, ought not to be counted among the living? Do we not need desperately, now, a vision which is capable of inspiring, of giving courage, of upholding every human being who is today involved in the next step towards our future? Such a vision must and can be for man to rise above the mere physical ground (whilst such a foundation is still with us); to rise into the new faith through knowledge while taking care that he does not rise into self-glorification or sink into escapism, or lack of will to do something about his future.

The Kingdoms of Nature and Beyond

This rising, this becoming master of both the tangible and the intangible world, is in the plan to attain total consciousness. Part of man's consciousness is, in fact, so beautifully captured in the animal, plant and mineral kingdoms that it is a most profound and joyous task for the human being to start releasing this into the total mind, reuniting all but this time on a conscious level; to protect the human being from the disaster of a completely mind-blowing experience and have a gradual dawning of which this being can be in full control. For that reason the division was made of the once total but unconscious state of paradise.

Through his capacity for thinking, intelligence and logic man can reason, deduce, enlarge or develop his consciousness. However, we as human beings cannot cope with an animal, plant or mineral consciousness without very clear and careful instructions, which is given in good meditation classes, courses, etc. The animal has a far wider field of sensitivity than man normally commands; it, however, cannot make deductions or intelligent use of this awareness. Instinctively it will either go to a place because a sympathetic kind of magnetism is driving it to go there or avoid a place by selecting an instructively perceived safer place. Animals are very aware of the ley line system of the earth; they know where positive and negative energies rule.

As we get to know all the kingdoms of nature we also suspect that there are kingdoms on the other levels and we begin to see that we are the link, that we were severed from this totality in order to get to know it. In this recognition development we will come to see that there is not one atom in matter that is not part of the whole, that each one of the atoms is, in fact, part of us and as we learn to love them we will be loved by them.

People who explore the world of the animal kingdom, such as Commander Cousteau, Joy Adamson, Gerald Durrell and many others, are making that link again with a consciousness which enlarges their own and that of their fellow men. Not one is left without this sense of wonder, awe and reverence; some of them I know personally and I feel awakened in me a tremendous sense of love and reverence towards the God who shines through their beings.

Others stretch out into the realm of the plant world where they become aware of the high level of sensitivity that quite surpasses the present human sensitivity. Marcel Vogel, Cleve

Backster and Dorothy Retallack, and many more, have all developed this high state of awe, for what they discover is the real entity they are dealing with then they involve themselves with that state of sensitivity of the plant kingdom.

If men without this new kind of understanding continue to think in their present confused and bewildered fashion, it is inevitable that a totally purposeless life will ensue. The cumulative effect of using drugs (LSD and to some lesser extent marijuana, hashish, etc.) is to break down man's thinking capacity and destroy his will-power. Plant and mineral consciousness is equally 'blocked' for man to begin with, and is only opened when a spiritual purpose is at the root of a human expansion of consciousness. Many indications of plant consciousness are described by Peter Tompkins and Christopher Bird in *The Secret Life of Plants* (Harmondsworth, Penguin, 1975).

The Lost, Ancient Wisdom

Wilhelm Karl von Gümbel, Teilhard de Chardin and Andrew Glazewski, to name just a few, were moving a stage deeper along the path of consciousness; they delved into the mineral kingdom where they found memories which are as yet completely unobtainable by man. The accuracy and refinement of the memory banks of crystals, metals and rocks are indeed realms which we must approach with awe and deepest wonder. What these souls discover is part of a world wisdom, deeply absorbed into this very foundation on which we so unthinkingly stand. The plumbing of this depth of total awareness is perhaps the key that will return us to the new paradise.

The following story, which will illustrate the kind of results obtained by a researcher of the calibre of Father Andrew Glazewski, happened on 22 November 1971. (Because music will be part of this book it is worth mentioning that this is the birth date of St Cecilia.) Father Andrew and myself visited the stones on the hills of the moor near Stover, he tuned into the stones by using delta waves and told me this tale from an age long past:

Here is a beautiful homestead; there were friendly people here, people who knew about healing and loving. Over there on the other side of that stone it is very dark [and he meant physical darkness, not the spiritual sacred darkness – let us call it anti-darkness]; they misused their knowledge, they did not listen with their hearts and even today they still hold this black magic spell. I would not go there if I were you [Father Andrew knew more than he could say]. One day we will have the power to help them to become free from their place of darkness which they created themselves, when we can free them through the power of love in the Christ being. Right over there [and he pointed to a place now very desolate] is another homestead; there are priests of a high order listening to the cosmic, preincarnated Christ who was teaching them then. They were given the understanding of fertility of seeds in plants, animals and man.

Some of this is related in *The Power of the Third* by Theo Gimbel (Hygeia Publications, Brook House, Avening, Gloucestershire 1975).

The fact that Father Andrew took me there was a great privilege which I shall not forget; we talked a lot about healing. That evening I was invited to speak at a gathering of a circle of his friends, and we concluded with a healing service in which he lovingly cleared the aura of those absent and present friends in need.

One thing the researchers mentioned earlier all have in common is that they develop a quality of humility which we all have to regain. Words to describe this are totally inadequate – even the word 'love' is not able to touch the real core of their attainment: trust, truth or submission and protection perhaps give us a slight understanding of their state of being. In other words, as we learn about these matters we are ourselves taken into the school of their teachings where we learn to be true servants of the universe.

The attitude of real listening (which was one of the skills considered essential by Andrew Glazewski, the listening and the real looking, allows those who really inquire and take the trouble to be taught to become the pupils of nature and to learn about their own selves. Teaching is, in short, nothing less than love: real love.

Many of the statements which will be found in this book may not be formulated in intellectually clear terms. Some of them cannot be expressed that way, and some are not meant to be intellectualised.

The many, sometimes completely unanswerable, questions must not be allowed to bewilder the reader. Rather let him say: leave it to my high consciousness for a while. In time the correct answer will come to all who seek the truth, as I have learned from my own experience.

Chapter 2

Dawning of Consciousness

Stages of Density Between Darkness and Form

When considering how we can help ourselves today, it is necessary to go back to the origins of matter. The manifestation of this planet passed through various stages, as shown in Figure 2.1.

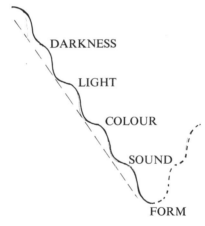

Figure 2.1 The stages of density between darkness and form.

DARKNESS AND LIGHT

Darkness is less dense than light.

I fully understand that in scientific terms darkness is not measured as an energy, because if we only measure light in relation to darkness we have nothing to measure darkness with. What follows that darkness? We touch on a very spiritual point here. And yet I must state, as many others have done, that darkness is an energy in its own right, or so my research has led me to conclude. I believe that from the point of total darkness starts a reversal of what we see when darkness turns into light. There is then a very high vibrational field that one might express as the 'inner light', inner colour, inner sound and form. We come into areas which have no space concepts anyway; but for us here in space and time we have to use the concepts we know. This concept we will find repeated later when we speak about the ductless glandular system of man.

COLOUR

Light, through the interplay with darkness, creates colour. Darkness is the original level of density from out of which sprang light. In the darkness even today the thoughts which we can conceive, when not asleep, are visions of an area which is usually protected by our sleep. After training, even in the monasteries and convents of the past and present ages, the fact that clearer thoughts and visions are possible at night is well known.

SOUND AND FORM

Colour sinks down into the lower vibratory rates and its next manifestation is sound. Sound is the powerful means by which form is created, first in the invisible state and then in the visible. Crystals are original sound forms. The 'singing orbs' which Shakespeare refers to in *The Merchant of Venice* are the original variations from which the visible world and man – and all that there is – have sprung. Rudolf Steiner speaks about sound *or* chemical ether, by which he reminds us of the very important link between chemistry and music. Furthermore, a metamorphosis such as colour into sound does not just happen through a gentle and gradual sliding downwards, but by a polarity action such as breathing in man, plant and animal.

Present-day science has discovered much but has by no means exhausted all the areas into which we are probing for answers. One of these areas is colour. The birth of colour, according to

Goethe (who was a very advanced scientist as well as a great poet), takes place through the interplay of light and darkness. That science cannot understand at present the finer and complex interaction of these two energies is just one more, as yet, unsolved area. My own present view is that we must investigate the areas of what we call shadow or twilight. Is it not as valid to speak of a degree of darkness as it is to measure a degree of light?

I am making here a plea to accept that darkness is an energy as much as light; and that the interaction of these two will, sooner or later, be understood more fully. .... In this world of man, the world of twilight and colour, we can find healing because colour is a phenomena that always appears at the edges where light and darkness meet. On this boarder experience is healing most effective; one can say it happens in the shadows of creation. Neither total light nor total darkness can maintain life. An open mind towards this area must be adopted. We must, as Steiner says, view with wonder that which we do not understand. With this attitude we will begin to be taught the secret workings of energies. Would we not die in either total light or total darkness? Total light would blind us; render us unconscious. In total darkness we tend to go to sleep, a sleep which eventually ends up in unconsciousness; if you like, death. Hence the area of colour is the healing force, the balance between the two extremes.

Some chemicals like water and oil do not blend under normal conditions. However when they are placed together and sound is used, molecular structure changes take place and the two will blend.

It is known that some extremely rare elements exist in the outer stratosphere which are not found on earth and also that these have a very short lifespan. In that realm where it is dark, because there is no light reflected, there is also sound which we cannot hear as it is so high on the scale of harmonics that it is inaccessible to the hearing capacity of any physical being. The wonders of creation may be manifested through the gradual slowing down of the vibrations. The darkness becomes light, the shadows colour, the colours sound, and sound creates forms. These forms become more and more durable and increase in their lifespan timewise; their chemical formulae stabilise; and by action and counteraction they learn to swing into movement, to breathe and ultimately to become a fine enough vehicle to be a dwelling for a soul and spirit.

The darkness here referred to is the primeval sacred beginning of all existence: in other words, the womb of creation. In this place life has its origin for us now. In healing work darkness will play an important part, as will be seen as we develop the concept of man. Out of this original state arises the next one, which stands in a complementary position to it – light. Light is denser than darkness and there are many ways in which this can be shown, even if this is very fine in actual physical terms; this is the next degree of density.

During the extensive experiments of Rudolf Hanschka, this scientist worked with one of the most sensitive pairs of scales in the world. He weighed the minutest quantities of wheat grains which would in a concealed ampule change in weight according to the moon phases. He noticed that light falling on one of the bowls would immediately register increased weight as against the one still in the shade.

Speed of Colour Vibrations

Blue light is less dense than red; red is the densest of all with a vibratory rate of 4.6×10^{14}, and blue with 7.5×10^{14}. (These figures can vary according to the very finest degree of colour and are here expressed in Herz. In English terms this is 630 billion, or 630,000,000,000,000.) It seems that because of the density, red is moving in its vibrational rate per second slower than blue.

If we divide the sum which lies between blue and red: $2.9 \times 10^{14} \div 8$ we will come to measurements which give us the whole visible colour range, as used in this book. (Just to give an idea of the speed of this vibration I suggest the following: take three fingers of one hand and call the thumb 1 million, each finger multiplies by 1,000, billion, trillion, and this is 10^{14}.)

Out of these two original complementary energies – darkness and light – arises the third which is colour. Colour is the subtle interaction between darkness (feminine) and light (masculine). Johann Wolfgang von Goethe was the first expounder in depth of a most useful theory of colour, which he wrote as far back as 1810. A number of useful books on colour have come out recently which are well worth reading if an understanding of colour in depth is required. (See book list, pp. 174–5.)

The next evolutionary swing into density is sound. It is at this point that involvement with the visible field begins. Moving from sightlessness to sight, and with sight then becoming enhanced by intensification of colour, we arrive at hearing. Sound has a formative energy; it actually produces beautiful sculptural forms. Its power is barely understood today. When sound comes into contact with air it vibrates this element into form. Furthermore, when sufficiently mobile particles are moved in the next denser element, vapour or mist, and finally in water, sound will create structures which are truly amazing.

In his institute in Switzerland, Hans Jenny has made a most extensive study of the reactions that sound has from liquids, iron filings, oils, sand and liquid plastics. Each sound, according to its pitch, changes the pattern, provided that the material is still mobile and in a state of flow. Hans Jenny has produced beautiful research results; so have Theodor Schwenk, John Wilks and Paul Schatz. When sound is used to co-orindate the finest matter we can see how in the womb of a physical being the new offspring is created. Ultimately sound touches densest matter and thus creates even mineral and solid rocks, steel, gold, etc. In this way we have arrived at solid form.

The initiate John, who contributed to the records of the life of Jesus of Nazareth who became Christ, puts this knowledge at the very start of his gospel: 'In the beginning was the Word and the Word was with God, and the Word was God.' He makes it abundantly clear that the point of impact of the invisible on the field of inert matter produces living matter, raising this to actual life – the point where visible man, animal, plant and stone appear. John the Evangelist takes the word, or the sequence of sounds which each word has, to explain that creation or arrangement of different connotations. Constellations in matter are raised according to the 'word sound' into the state of being, which is then constantly refined. He goes on to say 'And the light shineth in darkness; and the darkness comprehended it not'. If darkness would submit to light and would give up its existence to light we would no longer be conscious of light, nor could we live in such total light. One cannot stress enough the need to research into the significance of what is light and what is its 'sister' darkness. This is the most powerful of all the steps to be taken: implanting into matter the conscious God who has now the chance to raise this matter into eternal life. All diseases are due to the shortcomings of this raising to life of conscious man. How this is possible will be described in Chapter 3.

We can see how acoustics and optics arise from the growth of consciousness in man and how the whole field of physics is concerned with this planet's original solidification. Having now explained how this solidification took place, I would like to draw your attention to what the future must be. From the understanding of this awe-inspiring descent of man from God, we must shape a new vision of the ascent of man. The strongest possible means available to man today is love. Love in its fullest sense must reshape the lost vision. Jefferson's statement is so absolutely true: 'Without vision the people will perish.' If we are honest with today's world picture there is, for too many people, no true vision. We have almost succeeded in replacing it by material possessions such as a car, TV or refrigerator: what an appalling trinity! Buried in what could almost be described as the trashcan of our present society, we must rise from the banal and blasé attitude back to a man-as-God image. Restoring the divine dignity of each individual being is our duty and the only relevant way to follow on the path of healing.

The Etheric Sheath

Research means literally to *look again.* The depth to which we need to go when researching into this area eludes all of our present day electrical or mechanical instruments of recording or measurement, as the fineness is ultimately only recorded by the human sensitised, trained body and mental capacity. All visible things are surrounded by a greater area of measurable vibrations than we usually accept. Kirlian photography makes visible just a very narrow band of extra-sensory perception around plants, animals and man. This form of photography has originated from the work of two Russian scientists, Mr Sennyon and Mrs Valentina Kirlian. The technique is carried out with a high voltage generator using a photographic film. What is registered of living things, such as plants, animals and humans, is not just the physical outline and shape of the person or object, but also the finer electrical radiations which surround the object. These radiations, having nothing to do with electricity as we commonly know it, are circumscribed around the object but should not be confused with the actual aura, of which we will speak later. I should like at this stage to call it the 'etheric sheath'. This sheath does not stop where our comparatively clumsy physical instruments no longer register.

Telepathy is one of the few old phenomena which today survive even the general confusion of the highly sophisticated computer world. Where we rely totally on a manmade environment we also risk total breakdown of communication, which invariably paralyses whole enterprises. Then man, suddenly grappling in the dark, is thrown back on using the most complete instrument of all – the human body. This we must now research into and perfect again so that there is no breakdown. Human consciousness needs to grow and thinking capacity needs to be refined. This is not an intellectual rat-race but an expansion into a peaceful, relaxed and aware state in which we become so totally in touch that we can perceive even the finest of all vibrations.

Speed of Light and Thought Vibrations

I have mentioned the speed of colour vibrations; the next speed up is that of light. Most of us think this to be the ultimate speed but this is not so. It takes the sunlight 8½ minutes to reach us here on earth. You have already, at the mention of the word 'sun', sent your thoughts out to that ball of burning gas, and so we must accept that the speed of thought is faster than the speed of light, if not instantaneous. As soon as we come into contact with physical matter the speed of thought is impeded. The speed at which messages travel along the nerves of the human body and brain is measurable. This speed is no greater than that of light. (It varies with different types of nerves.) Yet man is in touch with the universe, not only with the moon, through the power of unimpeded thought.

According to Teilhard de Chardin, the creation of an image for the future of man is his own responsibility; but it is also a task in which he will need to re-co-operate with all the terrestrial and celestial energies. He will also need to learn how to do this out of complete freedom and without self-will or any egotistical motive.

Out of this material existence into which we have descended and where we exist in dusk of light, we will rise again into the dawn of light. Johan Wolfgang von Goethe in his publication *Zur Farbenlehre* (English translations called *Theory of Colour*), has drawn our attention to the evening and the morning colours which can be observed in such beauty. We are just emerging out of a cultural darkness: consequently we are experiencing the morning, the dawn colours. We also remember the colours of yesterday, yester-year even, and know that the whole world of colour is now opening up again. Mankind went through the stage of adolescence and is now a young, self-responsible and awakening adult. The rising out of this darkness of the world produces a challenge to science to reinvestigate the validity of colour in both its physical and its spiritual applications. Colour as a therapy is following music therapy, which is already an established help in medical treatment.

People such as Paul Nordoff, Clive Robbins, and Clive Muncaster are all working today in music therapy. Following in their footsteps in the field of colour are Hermann Proskauer, Roland Hunt, Professor L. Eberhard and Dinshah Ghadiali. Colour therapy means to help with – not to supplant – present medical work.

Man has taken hold of the material world and his ever deeper and closer identification with matter and the physical environment has produced a seemingly secure material outlook. Strangely enough, those who have finally integrated with this present stage of earth often find it necessary to look out and search into that which man once knew of the metaphysical, and what man also used as energies to build his world in the past.

If we were totally conscious beings we could benefit from far better health. To become conscious we must go back to the teachings which were once held in the temples. The master who brought these out into the wider world was Pythagoras. He himself underwent many changes during his early life. He was in touch with the Greek and Egyptian temple teachings. An account of his early years is given in Chapter 3. In the content of his thought the reader will find astonishing knowledge which was applied before and around 500 BC.

In Greece Pythagoras learnt the mastery of the soul, and in Egypt he learnt the discipline of the physical world. He lived in the astonishing time of change when the Egyptian teachings had almost died but still held important secrets. Then the light of Greece was rising in its most exalted teachings. People like Hippocrates, and later Plato, Sophocles, Aristotle and Archemedes, were masters of the philosophy of the heart. Archemedes was already on the brink of decline, using sacred laws for human intelligence – perhaps he is the father of technology. We must find our way back to Pythagoras and the teaching of the heart/balance energies.

The Eternal Spiral

Our aim is not to lead man to a reversal of time and its actions, but to rise through technology, to a real spiritual science which can use the technology as a foundation. The eternal spiral (see Figure 2.2) is our aim. We rise on the columns of our experiences. Starting at basic A1 we come to the next experience at B1 and move on from there to C1, only to arrive in time at A2, B2, C2 and A3, etc.

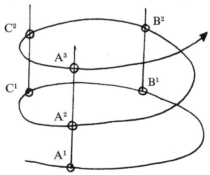

Figure 2.2 The Eternal Spiral.

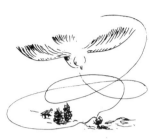

The energy which creates a spiral out of a circle is the energy of evolution. New heights and depths are found on the continuous path of a spiral. Orientation in space is one such new level of awareness. Birds orient their direction of flight by flying in a spiral when lost.

Chapter 3

Pythagoras and Hippocrates: The Forms of Past, Present and Future

'Pythagoras' is not a birth name, but the name given to an initiate. His seal (see Plate 1) is a most amazing reality of wisdom for which the animal is the snake (the human spine) and the measure of the field or given space. Four fields are, amazingly enough, also the chambers of the human heart. The upper two are the female and the lower two are the male chambers. Each half, however, contains elements of the other. The many secrets which are here dormant are inexhaustible. We will return to this in detail later in this chapter.

The Five Solids, the Four Temperaments and the Five States of Man

Hippocrates was born on the Greek island of Cos, which was a very important healing centre in antiquity. He is commonly styled the Father of Medicine. It is interesting that we find him defining four main types of man – the four temperaments as these are called – and it is important that we understand them. Rudolf Steiner refers to them in his educational works. What has not been considered is how Pythagoras adds to the understanding of man when we put Hippocrates' and his teachings together. The concept of the five states of man, as referred to in the following paragraphs, is greatly illumined when we consider the *five* Platonic solids (see Plate 4, between pages 84 and 93) in conjunction with the *four* temperaments. Each of these temperaments has inherent in it some of the elements of the other three.

In childhood we are always dominantly in one state, and the others are not expressed as firmly. The ideal state of the mature adult is to stand above, or say centred, and use all four states from the vantage point of the *fifth* position. The Platonic solid of the Pentagondodecahedron is placed as the balance in the centre. The sanguine personality is dominated by, or the centred person makes use of the Octahedron; the melancholic uses the Icosahedron; the choleric the Tetrahedron; and the phlegmatic person aligns with the Hexahedron. The connotations which accompany this are:

Pentagondodecahedron

Philosophy:	totality, the universe, etheric energies, archetypal harmony	
Mathematics:	total faces	12
	total edges	30
	total points	20
	angles of one face	108×5 (540°)
	angles of all twelve faces	6,480 (60×108)

Tetrahedron:

Philosophy:	fire, man; antennae* = hair	
Mathematics:	total faces	4
	total edges	6
	total points	4
	angles of one face	60×3 (180°)
	angles of all four faces	720 (12×60)

Octahedron:

Philosophy:	air, birds; antennae* = feathers	
Mathematics:	total faces	8
	total edges	12
	total points	6
	angles of one face	60×3 (180°)
	angles of all eight faces	1,440 (24×60)

Icosahedron:

Philosophy: water, reptiles; antennae* = scales
Mathematics: total faces   20
                   total edges   30
                   total points   12
                   angles of each face   60×3 (180°)
                   angles of all twenty faces 3,600 (60×60)

Hexahedron:

Philosophy: earth, mammal; antennae* = fur
Mathematics: Total faces   6
                   Total edges   12
                   Total points   8
                   Angles of each face   90×4 (360°)
                   Angles of all six faces   2,160 (24×90)

*The means by which final contact is made between the visible and the invisible environment.

To complete this description of geometrical form and mathematical order, relationship to man and man's relationship to the universe, we have now to take the average human breath rhythm per 60 seconds, which is 18, and see how this relates to the Platonic solids: 18×60 = 1 hour = 1,080 which is the radius of the moon in miles. Also, 108 is the atomic weight of silver, the metal attributed to the moon; 1080×24 = 25,920.

Let us go back now and see how the figures of the five Platonic solids fit into this figure, which incidentally is called the Platonic year, or the number of years it takes the sun to rise again at the spring equinox in the same place as, say, it did this year (although very slightly above the original point).

25,920 divided by

Dodecahedron	6,480 = 4
Tetrahedron	720 = 36
Octahedron	1,440 = 18
Icosahedron	3,600 = 7 + 720
Hexahedron	2,160 = 12

Inter-relationships

The inter-relationship between all the five regular solids becomes very clear when we consider the mathematical aspect of the angles. Angles have consciousness meanings. This is further enforced when these angles are used to construct the solids as named above. Each of these has specific qualities which can be used for therapeutic treatment of both psychological and health problems.

The five elements which are referred to here as being associated with these forms are part of the human body structure and its living tissue.

> *The Tetrahedron* representing fire is responsible for the warmth in the body of man. The temperature is vital to the health of all living matter.
>
> *The Octahedron* representing the air supports the breathing system of all the living environment.
>
> *The Hexahedron* supplies our structure in the skeleton and harder tissue matter down to metal and/or crystal such as diamonds.
>
> *The Icosahedron* is connected with all the fluid matter in the world around us.
>
> *The Pentagondodecahedron* is the life-conducting energy of the etheric field. This is in contact with the pineal and pituitary gland. Acupuncture is also in touch with these energies.

Antennae and the Environment

All physically visible things have a dividing surface between the inner parts and the air (already invisible) encircling them. Even the surface of a broken stone or metal starts from the moment of contact with air to form a skin made up of oxide that then will cover this newly exposed area. There is an interaction between all surfaces and the invisible. In animals and humans there is growth of hair, scales and fur. The nature of this is that it is a transmitter and receiver. What is received is always absorbed into the soul (psyche) and causes in animals and humans physical, emotional or consciousness reactions.

MANIC-DEPRESSIVES AND DEPRESSIVES

Manic-depressive humans act out destruction of their environment even to the point of killing. Many of our present-age man's reactions are manic-depressive, of a kind which are especially roused when exposed to an alliance such a human has made with a hero or team of football players. Then not only is failure or success of this hero absorbed via eyes or ears; the atmospheric conditions also spill over and are picked up by what we here like to call the antennae. Hair, when long in human fashions or cults, acts as a stronger antenna, and when it is short there is a blunting or shutting out of environmental messages.

The use of hair in cultures is a very important factor. Our culture has shown some awareness of this in the hippy movement, a softening and to some extent misused effect of this sensitivity. It is certain protection against sensitivity to environment when hair is cut short. In the middle ages, witches' hair was shorn as a punishment. Or women who wished to put the past behind them intuitively acted to aid this by cutting their hair. Good hairdressers can actually sense the health condition of their clients by the feel of hair.

We have now to turn to the condition complementary to that of the manic-depressive and consider the depressive personality. The antennae have received and transformed the received energy or messages into self-punishing and self-degrading, self-destructive actions – even leading to suicide.

In between these extreme states lie degrees of one or the other tendency. However, when the human being, by way of consciousness, determines the attitude to be in touch and has developed an awareness to use his sensitivity and let the antennae do the work in a controlled state of mental activity, then he can come to terms with a world that communicates by positive and meaningful messages being received, transformed and transmitted.

Plato, Aristotle and Pythagoras*

The fullest account of these thinkers is in *Rätsel der Philosophie*, Rudolf Steiner, Verlag der Rudolf Steiner, Nachlassverwaltung Dornach Schweiz 1914, which is not translated. Other books or courses contain only *references*, sometimes brief. Some of the most important are the following publications by the Anthroposophical Press.

* Information supplied by the Anthroposophical Society of Great Britain.

PLATO	(Hamburg) *Gospel of St John*, Lecture 9 *The East in the Light of the West*, lecture 3 *Genesis*, lecture 11 *Occult History*, lecture 3 *Wonders of the World*, lecture 7 *The* Bhagavad Gita *and the Epistles of St Paul*, lecture 7 *Karmic and Human Metamorphosis*, lecture 5 *Anthroposophical Life, Gifts*, lecture 10 (typescript)
ARISTOTLE	(Hamburg) *Gospel of St John*, lecture 10 *Gospel of St Luke*, lecture 3 *Genesis*, lecture 11 *Occult History*, lectures 3 and 6 *Wonders of the World*, lectures 9 and 10 *The* Bhagavad Gita *and the Epistle of St Paul*, lecture 1 *Secrets of the Threshold*, lecture 8 *Building Houses*, lectures 2, 3 and 8 *Background to the Gospel of St Mark*, lecture 3 *Menschliche und Mensch heitliche Entwick lungswahrheiten* (not translated), lectures 1, 2, 4 and 6
PYTHAGORAS	*The Gospel of St Matthew*, lecture 3 *Man in the Light of Occultism*, lecture 4 *Background to the Gospel of St Mark*, lecture 2

For information about the dates between which these thinkers lived, see Figure 3.1.

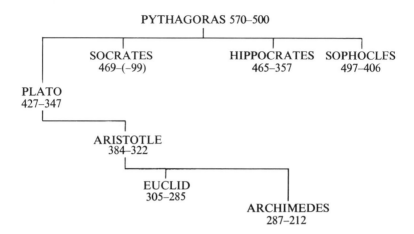

Figure 3.1 Chronological relationships between the greatest Greek thinkers (all dates are BC).

The Five Platonic Solids

The area of form is very important, not just because it is of healing value in supporting the colours, but also because of its value in a purely sculptural way. This sculptural element in form has the capacity to set up a change in the meaning of colour when it appears in another form. From our research we know that the perception of colour depends on the form in which this colour appears to the subject.

It is good to know some basic laws about form – after all we live in a world dominated by the shapes of the square and cube. Is this the best we can do? Are we in fact avoiding the issue of how to achieve a better environment for man? I would suggest that, far from considering the needs of man and then build, we consider only the economy of building; by and large, man still copes, but at the expense of his development in many cases.

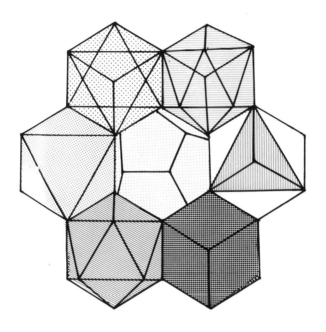

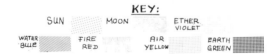

Using the most important grid of Hexagonal forms which appear in
basalt (staffa or other places) and the honey comb of bees or even
wasps, we can see that there is a basic energy to produce this form.
In the geometrical grid shown in this figure we can see as thinking
humans that both mineral and the 'un-blocked' insect obey universal
energy pattern.

The Ductless Glands

For the completion of the geometric table on page 40 we need to consider now the five Platonic solids in relation to the human body, especially to the main ductless glands.

Pentagondodecahedron: Pineal gland, totality and the gate to the whole universe. Also known as the crown. It is furthermore given the sense of touch in the body of man. A very fine symbol that can be placed in it also represents the wings of extraterrestrial beings. The thousand-petalled lotus flower.

Tetrahedron: Pituitary gland, also known as the third eye or brow. The gland that organises the bodily functions. Sense of sight. The two-petalled lotus flower.

Octahedron: The larynx or thyroid gland. The power of moving matter, healing. Also called the throat. Sense of hearing. The sixteen-petalled lotus flower.

The Cardiac Plexus: The heart, often also given the allocation to the sun energies. The true human wisdom lies in this centre of balance. The twelve-petalled lotus flower.

The Solar Plexus: In the region behind the stomach. Its capacity of responses to joy or sadness, anxiety or relaxation makes it akin to the waxing and waning of the moon energies. The ten-petalled lotus flower.

Icosahedron: The adrenal glands. The sense of taste. There is a mysterious link between this gland and the eyes. The beholding of the image in sight or the remembering of the genetic pattern seem to have a real connection with each other. The six-petalled lotus flower.

Hexahedron: The sacral gland. The root or base. The sense of smell (scent). The four-petalled lotus flower.

Apart from these seven glands there are numerous others which are distributed throughout the human body. However, those listed above give a picture of the principle that lies behind the human body, which is not just a physical apparatus. Throughout our work we must become ever more mindful of the vast secrets which are still unrevealed but can dawn gradually in our minds as we inquire deeper into this field of total relationship: that nothing is separate; that everything is related to the whole.

The Number 25,920

The first six numbers in units 1, 2, 3, 4, 5, 6, when arranged in a particular way, produce between them the number 25,920 as follows:

2^6 (two to the power of six)

3^4 (three to the power of four)

5^1 (five to the power of one)

$= 64$
$= 81 \quad (64 \times 81 \times 5) = 81 \times 64 = 5,184 \times 5$
$$= 5 = 25,920$$

It is also noteworthy that all Platonic figures are divisible by 9 and/or 3.

Why, we may ask, does the Icosahedron not adhere to this law? Because man is not a separate being from the earth or water. More than four-fifths of man is liquid and in terms of humidity the earth is also far more water containing than what we normally accept. So, all is interwoven, solid, liquid, rhythm and form of which also the human breath is a part.

Ideal Balance and Health

Now we may once more go back to our consideration of the four temperaments and see how there arise four states of imbalance and one state of ideal balance in man's capacity for health. The task of healing is to compensate for these imbalances, so that a true human being can stand in the state of ideal balance. On the life path, all people experience each one of these states of imbalance at a certain level. However, we are here concerned with the pathological condition. All the nervous breakdown cases can be generally grouped around these four temperaments, or types. We can illustrate this as follows. We have, broadly speaking, three main perception levels on which we operate as conscious people in everyday life. Perception of our environment is the first-level 'intake'. The second is that we measure the intake against previous experiences, offer an objective assessment which contains also logic and reason, an accommodating of the intake. This we may call 'balance'. Out of these two we then decide to take our next step: this we call 'action'. In the last drawing we can see three planes: the door plane, the table plane and the wheel plane. The door plane is intake, the table plane balance, and the wheel plane we call action.

In normal life (which does not exist at all) we would find these planes tending all the time towards adjustment to each other. In this way we progress on our daily path fairly well. Let us call this Stage V. When this smooth co-operation between these three planes of consciousness becomes impaired, then the personality of the human being suffers a nervous breakdown in four different directions.

Say that the intake (door plane) collapses and becomes identified with the table plane (balance) and the action plan identifies also with this table plane, then we have a total nervous breakdown into the depressive personality. This then becomes Stage I.

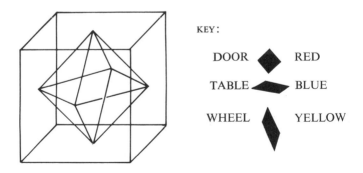

Figure 3.2

The next possibility is that the intake and balance planes identify themselves with the action plane, and thus we will have a manic-depressive nervous breakdown – Stage II.

When the balance plane and the action plane identify with the intake plane, the nervous breakdown position becomes a violent type, a psychopath – Stage III.

Finally, the three planes can freeze into immobility and the person is in the static pathological condition – Stage IV.

In case history, it is almost always confirmed that the four breakdown conditions are related to the original bias of the person in whom they occur.

Stage I   Melancholic
Stage II   Sanguine
Stage III   Choleric
Stage IV   Phlegmatic childhood
Stage V   Well-educated culturally, not necessarily
            intellectually

Architecture

Having examined the Platonic solids, we now have to find how form as such can influence man in his health pattern. It is not immaterial in what kind of environment man lives, works, rests and plays. Ultimately it is vital for him to be subjected to form which can help in the healing process (see Table 3.1). Any one of the pure regular solids produces in man a most definite impression. We have come from the round hut, the igloo, to the square, perhaps tentlike structure, but soon developed the pyramid (octahedron).

Not only the human mind, but also human physiology is affected by form. To live in a pyramid or to work in it was never intended. As we know, energy is made available by the enclosing space (see Wilhelm Reich's work on orgone energy). What the pyramid really was will only be understood if we reckon with these energy levels raised by its amazing form. The outside walls, all four of them, were used as a radar screen of quite unique capacity. Each culture has its own architecture

TABLE 3.1   CORRELATION CHART OF THE EFFECTS OF THE FIVE REGULAR SOLIDS

	TETRAHEDRON *Red*	OCTAHEDRON *Yellow*	HEXAHEDRON *Green*	ICOSAHEDRON *Blue*	PENTOGONDO- DECAHEDRON *Violet*
COLOUR	Red	Yellow	Green	Blue	Violet
PSYCHOLOGICAL EFFECT	Claustrophobic, collecting, stimulating	Expansion into timelessness	Logical abstract, security-holding and orientation	Flow, restlessness, in touch with many levels of perception	Harmonising and **enlivening**
PHYSIOLOGICAL EFFECT	Energising, speeding up of body rhythms	Hyperventilation	Reducing body rhythms, hardening	Softening of body tissue, dissolving structure	Synchronising of body rhythms
THERAPEUTIC USE	Gathering, concentrating, recovering self-awareness	Reducing introverted personality, detachment with direction, tension-inducing	Physically balancing, enclosing in a secure space, removing fear, anchoring and increase of tension	Remobilising of psycho- and physiological patterns, removing obsessional ideas and behaviour patterns, reducing tension	Raising of dignity and self-respect, balancing out manic-depressive and depressive states of mind
MATHEMATICAL SPACE PROPORTIONS	$\dfrac{H \times B}{2} \times 8 = S$	$\dfrac{H \times B}{2} \times 8 = S$	$H \times B \times 6 = S$	$\dfrac{H \times B}{2} \times 20 = S$	$A + A_7^1 \quad \dfrac{H \times B}{2} \times 24 = S$ $+ C \quad \dfrac{H \times B}{2} \times 12 = S_7^1$ $S + S_7^1 = S$
ANGLE SUMS AND PLATONIC YEAR	$36 \times 720 = 25,920$	$18 \times 1,440 = 25,920$	$12 \times 2,160 = 25,920$	$7 \times 3,600 + 720 = 25,920$	$4 \times 6,480 = 25,920$

Provided all edges of the five solids are identical, the surface area will be increased as follows:

Key: H = Height $\dfrac{H \times B}{2} \times 4 = S$
  B = Base
  S = Surface
  S = Total Surface

and thereby accumulates the energies for the leaders of these cultures: às if all four sides of this structure, which helped man to anchor to the earth, were ears to listen to the universe, the triangular surfaces were oriented towards the four points of the compass.

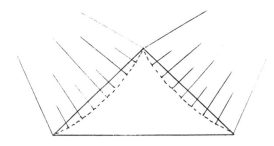

Figure 3.3 Pyramid Concavity. The very slightly concave sides of the pyramids are actually very vast radar screens which show that the ancient people knew an art which we have re-discovered on another level. With it they 'sensed' part of the universal vibrations.

The human being of today needs other energies. The Egyptians had to become earth-bound. The pyramid was ideally suited to their style of life. In the Greek cultural epoch man developed a new style which was taken beyond its time into the building of the cathedrals and churches. The square, and out of it the rectangle and cube, or double cube, arose. The cube is the dual of the octahedron. The age of technology seems to have brought about the development of a cubic architecture which very few people really like. We are today dominated by this form, but it has shut us into the space. Just as the pyramid is a mind-blowing and time-removing energy today, for man's consciousness is changing, so has the cube the effect of imprisonment and a hardening of his being. Out of these two forms is created one overwhelming mental stimulus, which the initiate priest could use, but most lay people cannot make head or tail of. The cube actually creates the opposite effect — a dulling and a darkening of man's higher perception.

Out of this we now need a new architecture. The use of the icosahedron could produce (and there is evidence of this) a human mind which has lost its anchor and floats aimlessly into the endless waters of the world. Nor does the tetrahedron give us the space we need and it would stifle us in a pressure of tremendous heat. This is not yet an established fact, but stands a good chance of being proved true, considering the knowledge we have about the other spaces.

This leaves us with the pentagondodecahedron. Even though this is the body of totality, it would need artistic modifications to be really useful for pure living space. It is most recommendable for healing, as our research has shown.

The most successful redesign of a living and healing environment is a modification of the severity of the 90° angle, so much over-used today. We have called it the triangular conversion (see plate 5 between pages 84 and 93). This conversion helps the human being who is inside such a space to be in a harmonious and protective environment. The squareness and hard corners are transmuted and space becomes more agreeable. Have we not seen this conversion in Victorian ceiling embellishments and earlier architecture? Chartres, the spiritual school from 1280 to 1350, was perhaps the most powerful spiritual centre in Europe. Thomas Aquinus, one of the outstanding teachers there, knew of the ancient healing and teachings of the Greek temple secrets, and the need to translate such knowledge, as Pythagoras did, into the acceptable terms of his day.

Steiner, in a way, created a new school of spiritual science in Switzerland. At Dornach two buildings were erected to house this school. The first, made of wood, burnt down in 1922; the second, made of concrete stands today in the same place and is, like the first, called Goetheanum.

If the cathedral at Chartres has an amazing amount of the sacred geometrical designs, proportions, laws and measurements, the first Goetheanum had all the principles of this incorporated, an as yet unrepeated achievement. This is healing architecture and we must try to study it so that at least some of its art can be used for healing today.

Architecture was always based on the measurements of man; thus we can now look at man from the view that this 'house' is also the principle of architecture for the future. Pythagoras was aware of these laws and we today are in need of recovering these for our progress.

The Seal of Pythagoras

On 21 June 1971, at 3 a.m. in Attingham Park, Shrewsbury, England, Sir George T., Ruth B., Basil H. and myself were left in the eighty-bedroom house; 220 guests who stayed there for a weekend had left late that afternoon. With some blackcurrant juice – as if there was nothing else in the house – we four celebrated the summer solstice. For the first time it was possible to have a long talk to Ruth, who was the personal secretary to Sir George.

Midnight had long passed and I was sleeping, or rather not sleeping, in the dark room next to Ruth's. I told her of some old experiences of many years past. Now in the silence and darkness of the night came and went the faces, some crying, some smiling, and time and again that very special face which had come several times before – I can always remember the dates when it has appeared. So far it has happened three times in my life. Then I was looking down. Below me lay a valley and in it was a garden; in this garden were four squares, absolutely exact squares with hedges of deep green – no, as I looked, these hedges were black, they were not hedges at all, they were the body of a black snake that had laid itself around this garden, dividing it into the four squares.

I remembered the vision. I wrote it down later and had very little idea of what it actually was. About a year later I was speaking to a friend who has considerable knowledge of the Greek mysteries. I drew the vision for her again and found that she was able to translate it for me. She simply put against the snake 'Pytha', and against the field 'Agoras'. From this I have realised that this was the seal of the master Pythagoras (see plate 1 opposite p. 84). Through this experience I have learned much.

The seal also depicts the heart with its four chambers. Again, if we have the law 'as above so below' (as in the universe so also in the atom), we can say that the heart represents a whole human being; without doubt the principles are there. In the upper two chambers are represented the two energies of both the dark (used) blood and the light (rejuvenated) blood from the lungs. In the lower two chambers are placed the next stages: to the lungs, where it is oxygenated; from there it returns as new blood into the left auricle and down the left ventricle and from there into the body, returning in due course to the right auricle to complete the cycle.

Man in the present state is a duality, in as much as the two energies of man and woman are polarities that work together, complementing each other and creating a third energy.

The Heart

We can represent the heart by the design shown in Figure 3.4. Blood with toxins is brought into the right auricle A^1; then given to the right ventricle B^1; then it passes through the lungs into the left auricle B^2; and from there into the left ventricle A^2. This means that both right chambers of the heart have blood which we could call 'mature' with experience, and the left side of the heart has 'virgin' blood to take back to the body.

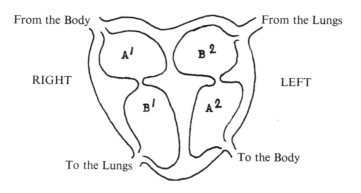

Figure 3.4 The heart.

Male/Female Polarities

If we now take it that the woman represents the intuitive aspect of the human being, she nevertheless has aspects of both male and female within her; consequently, A and B energy. These will be the auricles of the heart. The man (male) has the practical tasks, the logical function of taking mature blood to the lungs and virgin blood to the body again; he also has both aspects, B and A. We can now say that the auricles are representing the woman and the ventricles the man, each being a certain totality on their own but creating a bigger capacity of free association, sharing each other's polarities. Interestingly we have reversed polarities in each so that the co-operation is more effective than it could possibly be without this reversal.

If we return to the seal of Pythagoras we can understand why this master was the greatest teacher of his day. further, we may now look into the future where we might see this master playing a significant role; for his teachings of old are still relevant to our needs of today and tomorrow.

It will be noted that the word which can be read from this design and seal is ABBA, which is the ancient word for the Father. The snake, the beast of protection, is keeping in safe custody the jewels, the fields of the father ground. When Buddha found total illumination he woke up the snake (dragon) to enlighten for him the centre which is known as the *kundalini* power. We also see now how man is related by the master Hippocrates to the four elements of nature. He saw great depth in all the human physical and mental states, we can again find this orientation to the four elements which offers the possibilities for the fifth, the Ether.

Let us consider once again the five Platonic solids and the four physical elements. We see that we need to acknowedge the existence of the invisible and inaudible fields as well as the human states. Hippocrates' four temperaments are simplifications of the human being in the round: a good actor takes up the part of the dancer, the sanguine; the psychologist is more a melancholic; the down-to-earth, practical man, choleric; and the thinker, the phlegmatic. But he who is fully a man is also in command of any these capacities at the time of need for 'acting a role'.

The four temperaments form two pairs: earth and water are horizontally placed at our feet and reflect the melancholic and phlegmatic humours. Fire and air are upright, less dense than the other two, and are sanguine and choleric in character (see Figure 3.5). Thus we could say that intuitive, more feminine characters are the latter. But in the ancient symbolism we find fire–male, air–female, water–female and earth–male identifi-

45

cations. Thus again we have a wonderful polarity in this image. Each is both a completeness and a polarity. The mobility and flexibility of water and wind display the intuitive nature of woman. The fire of thinking – light – together with the logical structure of earth (rock) are male attributes.

Hippocrates relates male to fire and air and woman to water and earth. There are cross-references to be made all the time, as man is the most mobile of all creatures.

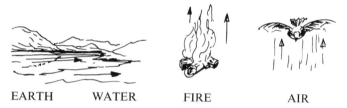

EARTH   WATER   FIRE   AIR

Figure 3.5 Horizontal and upright characteristics of the elements.

Metamorphosis on the Theme of the Double Helix, the Heart and the Human Energies

The double helix has in the human being come to be a most perfected exchange of energy. In each inter-reaction there is not only a flow and return flow, but also a spiral effect on each of the enclosed points (see Figure 3.6).

Artists sometimes produce designs such as the one shown in Figure 3.7 by drawing on memory at the very deepest, unconscious level. This is in fact a symbolic energy line, and such lines will often be found to follow variations of the figure 8. The heart has a double figure 8, which points to its uniqueness as well as function as the eternity symbol. Other such energy lines can be seen in the human body when one considers the positioning of eyes and breasts, adrenals, kidneys and ovaries (or testicles). The figure 8 also appears in molecular structures.

Through the natural influences of life in co-operation with the elements these most beautifully aligned currents, creating invisible flow and counterflow spirals, may, on becoming visible (and therefore this distorted to a greater or lesser degree) produce their own kind of asymmetrical beauty. This form of living beauty is more acceptable than dead, accurate symmetry.

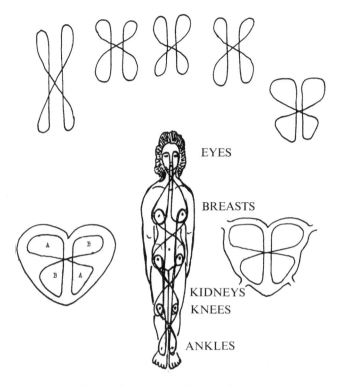

EYES

BREASTS

KIDNEYS
KNEES

ANKLES

Figure 3.6 The double helix in the human being.

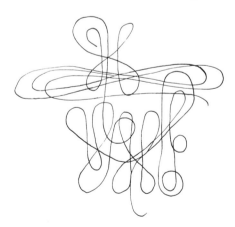

Figure 3.7

Chapter 4

Light and Colour as a Physical, Psychological or Spiritual Science

From time immemorial colour has been a great medium for art and, until the thirteenth to fourteenth centuries, art was the prerogative of religions all over the globe. In the Western world the Church held great power over the trades and arts alike and thereby the guilds of craftsmen were obliged to treat their knowledge as part of the gift of God. Apprentices were trained very slowly and took years to acquire the deeper knowledge of their craft. Some of the craftsmen, such as dyers and painters, were finally sworn into the guilds; this meant that the trade secrets were not to be given to anyone except those who were made fellows of that guild. Today there are no such limitations and one has the benefit of going, as a lay person, into shops to purchase any colour, dye or coloured filter.

Colour in Daily Life

Some people know which colour to use for what purpose and others do not. Some have even learnt to use colours to manipulate their fellow humans into certain actions to profit from this knowledge. Others are looking at colour as a pretty decoration which they judge to be aesthetic. Very few actually use colour in order to help their fellow human beings to better living and health.

Colour can be applied as a pigment to walls, dresses, pictures, crockery and a thousand other things. It can be used as light, but this is far less frequently done and very little is known of the results of using coloured lights. Here at the Hygeia Research

Studios we have become much more aware of the use of colour and can actually predict what coloured lights will do to people, animals and plants. In the appendix are several special research papers which give some insight into this very effective use of colour.

It is possible to use colour by simple thought projection and effectively send it to any distance, provided the techniques by which this is done are fully known. I will describe in Chapter 6 some practical experience in this field.

The chemical make-up of an individual seems to depend on the release of the chemicals from the nerve ends into the body. Each one of us is a separate being, although also a member of a race, tribe, clan or family. The individual directs through his or her being the rate and speed of the release of these chemicals. Furthermore, the movement of these fine substances can be accelerated or retarded by sound and colour. Any sounds a person hears work gently on these changes. Sounds sung or words spoken by a person have a much stronger impact upon this individual's chemical changes, especially mantras repeated regularly, which can bring about very decisive changes. An example of a 'heard' sound is your given name, which works upon you all your life and, therefore, this name is important.

Colour has an even deeper impact upon man. It is like a medicament in homeopathy, where the higher potencies have a more powerful impact in the healing. Colour, being a much higher vibration than sound, has consequently a stronger impact upon the human being, or any living substance. Thus even finer chemical changes are effected by colour than by sound.

It must be understood that most dress materials, with a very few exceptions, act as colour filters. To the extent to which the body is covered, the body receives a colour treatment. This is usually a personal choice. Women more than men choose a colour intuitively and this colour may be worn through a whole phase of their lives, or only occasionally. The reason why women are more aware than men is because their bodies, and consequently their minds, are less deeply steeped in the mineral density; therefore a sensitivity is still prevailing in them which the density level in men does not permit.

Provided that there were sufficiently accurate and sensitive instruments to measure the truth of above statement, we would come to this conclusion scientifically. Furthermore, it would not be surprising if in archeology male bones were found of more ancient periods than female bones. This is at the moment not proved, but the chances would be high. On the emotional level a woman is more responsive and reacts to colour much more quickly than a man (see our research in Chapter 7). The above findings are from the Hygeia research into human environment and we are certain that it will not be long before another research project substantiates our findings.

The Qabalah

At this point it would be interesting to look at the Qabalah, an ancient and well-proven system, according to which the Jews were able to rise to a highly cultural, economical and intelligent level of life. In this system the two halves of man are depicted as being the interplay of two halves of one whole.

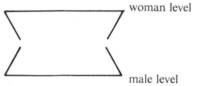

woman level

male level

The woman, being attached more to the intuitive awareness and psyche, finds herself based not so much on the here and now as on the more eternal level, with a wider, albeit not so easily definable, accurate perception but the need to come to terms with the daily physical environment, taking her two-sided being A⟷B down to make contact with the world of matter, the capacity to materialise energy. A is the original spiritual capacity and B is the vessel-making, raising of physical matter into the visible world. So A and B must work together in order to have the result C.

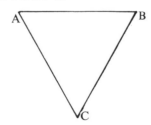

The male task is quite different from the woman's needs, and can be said to contain the strong B energy at one end and the A energy at the other B⟍——⟍A. The vessel is manifested (B) and indicates the striving towards the original source, the spiritual link. C becomes then the aim which is to achieve the point completely complementary to the woman.

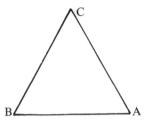

Only when this is completed are we in the presence of MAN, that being who is neither male or female, but has achieved the being that stands above sex: division. When this is achieved a very important stage of human evolution will be completed. We can say that at that point we would return to the state which was pre-matter, namely, sound. The Christ has attained this stage and therefore is not bound to the matter of physical properties, but, from this point of view, has achieved the return or the rising into the world of sound or chemical ether; according to Rudolf Steiner there will again be the sound, the word, creative and human (etheric) beings capable of creating off-spring by pure sound.*

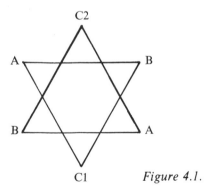

Figure 4.1.

* See also Theo Gimbel, *Key, Lock and Door*
Hygeia Publications, Brook House, Avening, Glos.

51

'Colour Hue'

There are few people who have perfect pitch. This can partly be trained through constant practice of music. A person with this gift can name a sound on hearing it. This ability is not yet known to exist widely for colour, but it is a possibility which many people could be trained to attain. Very few people at present have a perfect 'colour hue', which is what one could call this. Most people go to a shop and memorise a colour which they think they would like to match. I know of only a few who could accurately measure the colour seen in two different places over a period of time. There are some people who can do this just as there are people with perfect pitch. It is a rare gift but does exist.

The many substances used for the dyeing of cloth and the glazes in ceramic work are highly delicate and have, from time immemorial, been known to be very difficult to repeat accurately when one particular lot of glaze or dye has to be remade.

Colouring media used in ancient Egypt

(a) TO BE USED ON GLASS

dark blue	cobalt
light blue and green	copper/green: iron
yellow	antimony and lead mixture
rose-gold	gold mixed with small quantity of iron
red	copper oxide

(b) TO BE USED FOR PAINTING (pigment colours)
Except for black, all colours were of mineral origin.

black	soot with powdered charcoal as a fixing agent; resin from trees
white	chalk or plaster (heated alabaster)
red	red ochre; iron oxide
dark yellow	yellow ochre derived from iron oxide-hydrate

light yellow   sulphurarsen (arsensulphide)
                                      covered with beeswax

Shadows

We are less aware of colour when it comes to shadow colours.
Most people put them down as grey or black, but careful
observation shows that this is not the case. We can do the
experiment shown in Figure 4.1 quite easily.

A is a torch
A1 is a coloured filter used during the experiment
B is a second torch
B1 is a second coloured filter
C is an opaque object, possibly a vase, jug or piece of
   cardboard
D is a screen or white wall, or a piece of white cardboard
   20in×30in

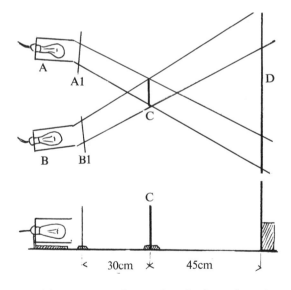

Figure 4.2 Apparatus for testing shadows for colour.

Switch on torch A and Black out the rest of the room. Object
C will now throw a shadow on the white card. After having

looked at this shadow, place a screen of cinemoid or theatrical jell (A1) in front of the torch and look again at your shadow. Let us suppose your colour filter is red: the shadow will take on a dark green colour. Now to enhance this experiment take another torch (B) and place it a foot away at the same level as A with another coloured filter. Now there will be two shadows, one for each torch. One shadow will now not be the same green but will have changed in accordance with the colour filter of the second torch. Suppose it was blue; your shadow will now be orange and the green shadow will have turned turquoise. (*Fig. 4.2*)

It is worth noting that these coloured shadows are colours which are very clear and delicate; they have an almost ethereal quality. Those who can see aura colours will connect this quality with the phenomenon quite easily. Coloured shadows are the corresponding effects which are the harmonics of sound. Just as in sound, overtones and harmonics are most helpful in healing, so, in colour, are the shadows. The instrument which we call the 'colour composer' relies on this factor.

If we incorporate a colour wheel, which is used for the blending of the eight degrees of hues in the eight main colours, in the experiment, we can take, say, a blue which is leaning towards the turquoise, another of the middle range and a further one of the violet range. Still using our shadows we can now get from the three different blues a total range of colour, in as much as we will have a reddish shadow, a greenish shadow and a yellowish one. This simple experiment will show you what a wide range each colour has when we allow the spectrum to be used together with the shadow colours.

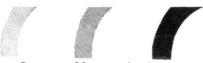

Degrees of hues and colours.

A further experiment ought to be made so that the student in colour therapy becomes really familiar with a phenomenon which again we are mostly not aware of. Take a brightly coloured object and look at it for between a quarter and half a minute; then turn your gaze on to a white surface and wait to see what will appear there. What you will see is even clearer and closer to the aura colours. The original object, if it was yellow, will now appear in a violet colour. Try the same experiment looking at a dark grey or matt black surface instead of white. Our eyes are wonderful instruments which continually balance out in our vision what we see in colour. The arrangement of rods and cones in the eye is highly sensitive and responds to colour very much more than we think. The colour you see after this experiment is called the after-image. It fades out if the eye is not re-stimulated with any particular colour. However, when you have been in a room that has been flooded with a particular coloured light, either daylight through stained glass or theatre floods with filters, you will, on leaving this area, be facing the complementary colour. Some people are so sensitive to colours that they have to be considered carefully before they are exposed to them. It is often in such cases good to use very delicate colours at first and then progress to deeper shades.

In his advise for people with weak eyes, Rudolf Steiner suggests using the following:

> An 8in disc is painted in blue on a large sheet of paper: leaving a good gap of 14 to 16in and paint a red disc of similar size. Hang this up at eye-level and let your eyes soak in the blue colour. After half a minute, take your eyes off the blue and put them on the white in the middle. Let the after-image gradually fade out, which will take about quarter of a minute. Now fixing your eyes on the red disc and soak in this colour; return to the white and then, when the after-image has faded, back to the blue. Do this about three times ending with the blue. This will greatly strengthen the eyes, especially if you have had any eye strain.

Colour-Blindness

Here we should also discuss colour-blindness. There are predominantly three areas: one is total absence of colour perception and the person can only see shades of grey, white and black; another is the group of red/green reversal; and there is a further group of yellow/blue confusion. These are not serious problems as there is usually some compensation – a very good brain for mathematics, excellent general memory capacity and an ability for good concentration. Strangely, colour still has the expected impact on the colour-blind person. The reaction is the same as if the sight was so-called normal.

Finally, what about totally blind people? Some of these people are, in fact, far more colour-sensitive than the sighted person, and it is an absolute fallacy to think that, because they cannot see, their environment is unimportant. When we subject blind people to coloured light their reaction is the same as those who are sighted. Can these people be trained to recognise colour? The answer is yes, they can be helped to do this.

It is said that our hands, particularly our palms, are extensions of our brain. We do not use our hands or fingers usually for any other purpose except to take hold of things and to move objects. This is not the sole purpose of the human hand. In fact latent in all people are capacities which we never use unless life has pushed us into an alleyway where they are required. I have been shown at an Institute for the Blind in Boston Watertown, Massachusetts, by the Rev. Lesley Price, how blind people are trained to 'see' colour.

Place a red flannel about 1ft square on a table and next to this a blue one. Put one hand on each. The blue one will seem to be receding from us, whilst the red, as it were, pushes into us. This can be picked up by the palms of blind people much more readily than by sighted people. When the blind student has been able to register the difference, the flannels are changed over and finally shuffled at random. The hands of the blind do not touch the flannels but are some 2 to 3in away, hovering above the flannels. When the students have become sure of the difference, one of the flannels is replaced – maybe the red is now a yellow one. The student now learns more quickly and will soon pick up the difference. Later green, orange and violet flannels will be recognised and the student begins to take notice of the dresses the staff wear and what colour the curtains are. I was once told by a blind person: 'You are wearing some blue and there is another colour also but I can't "see" it; there is too little of it.' I opened my jacket and asked 'What is the other colour?' 'Oh now I see – it is yellowy.' (It was a gold-coloured sweater which I exposed to the girl.)

The student who works with colour therapy will soon find that there are areas which we cannot put into the limitations of a book and that colour does not conform to the scientifically foolproof experiments which can more easily be done with the lower density of sound. The completely accurate perception and reaction to colour in each individual depends on the chemical protein basis upon which the person builds his or her whole health pattern. Whilst there is a wide range of agreement, there are nevertheless very marked differences which come to the fore when we try and work with sound and colour compatibility.

Sound, as has been demonstrated by the work of Hans Jenny, can show us the very definite scientific way in which it works; colour has still to be linked with what we call the accepted view of the present world. However, colour is so much less dense than sound that there are greater difficulties to overcome if we try to understand how very accurately and extraordinarily diverse this area of our world is. For each individual human and the members of the animal kingdom it is possible to identify an increasingly precise hue of colour that is associated with each. In Chapter 6 we shall refer to the need to offer an adjustment to the wide range of hues which are selected by the sub- or super-consciousness of each being. Whilst there is blue that calms and red that stimulates, there are precise degrees of each hue that will affect one person more than another. Thus we realise that we can use colour as a therapy but also that we must allow for individual adjustment. The broody hen has chosen the red laying box almost without exception over years of observation. The blue box was sought out by all others at random and the neutral one was also used on and off. This is only a very loose day-by-day observation which I have made while feeding our hens. Colour also plays a part in plant growth: see Appendix I.

Colour and the Ductless Glands

It is known that the blue has a much faster vibratory rate than red, and yet blue is the colour in which we relax, red the colour which brings excitement.

The body of a human being incarnates into this earthly environment, or shall we say that the human soul calls together, the energies which hold the power over the substances which produce a body here visibly on earth. From this point of view we must regard the *pineal gland* as the most important ductless gland. This has, as a colour, a very fine distribution of magenta. It is the gland responsible for translating the invisible energies into visible energies.

The colour spectrum sinks down from ultra-violet (magenta) out of the invisible band of this vibration, through the visible world of sense perception, until finally it disappears into infrared. The human being is a column of light and vibrates into this visible world by picking up the law of colour and playing, sounding to the rhythms of both these areas, before and during the stages of being a manifest body – having a visible entity for an average of seventy-two years. According to the old traditions of both the Western and Eastern cultures, there is wide acceptance of the fact that all manifested beings have a vibrational field that condenses through the range of the spectrum and sound scales. The reader should accept this idea as possible, and use the thoughts stimulated by this concept to draw conclusions. We should never discard an idea on first hearing, or discovering it for ourselves, but keep an open mind.

Here is what years of research have found to work out well for a vast number of people.

The very fine colour of magenta is also described by Rudolf Steiner as the colour of peach blossom. I mention this here because it is this exquisitely fine and gentle colour that seems to give rise to the chemistry of man being stimulated into interreaction with the elements of the earth. In the Indian tradition this is the crown *chakra* (gland). In the human brain this lies slightly behind and above the pituitary gland which is associated with the colour dark blue. In Western tradition it is called the brow or the third eye. This gland then takes over the organisation of the elements raised by the crown gland.

Medically it is accepted that the pituitary gland has the capacity to conduct its messages throughout the human body and by this co-ordinate and uphold the image of health in the body. The third eye is the place where we make the mental image of what we are told and cannot physically see there and then. Hence, also, image making is a vital part of health preservation.

The *pineal gland*, which is not usually regarded as important in medical investigation, is nevertheless the gland which offers access to a path that links man to the invisible world, and it is therefore vital to our survival. When that gland is not working at all in man, then gradually our life energies ebb away until the body dies for lack of nourishment through spiritual food. There are many accounts of people who have survived most unacceptable states of existence because of their belief in what we call spirit or God. The pineal gland is constantly translating the necessary energies from the invisible into the visible, from where the pituitary gland is actually ordering the rhythms. The rhythm of breath and heart beat and the rhythm of our sexual glands are all being beautifully co-ordinated through this second gland. Next below is the *thyroid gland*, or the throat. This is associated with the colour turquoise. As the centre of sound it plays an important part in the well-being of man, who needs to balance his body. Sound has the capacity to change the chemicals in the body, or, better, the opportunities are given to create a fusion of two chemicals. By the regular use of a particular sound or sequence of sounds, the body can obtain both mental and emotional and also physiological changes. It is interesting to record here some personal experience I have had.

After the Second World War, I was a captive of the Russian Army and found myself in the region of South Ural for three and a half years, imprisoned with five thousand men. Many died because of the lack of knowledge of how to retain a bond between the spiritual and the physical, though we may call it starvation. I remember at the end of two years' captivity we were able to hear for the first time a very roughly made violin played by a professional player. I and a large number of others sat on the bunks listening. Tears were running freely down the cheeks of many. This first 'concert' led to the combining of several who were musicians in the camp. More violins and accordions were built. (The first accordion was so heavy it had to be stood on a little stool in front of the player.) This led us to remembering operas, writing them down on cement bag paper. Each time we rehearsed, more was remembered. Finally, the whole of *Aida* was put together. As there were no women to sing the female parts, young men rehearsed and played the parts of women. In the course of one year these young men

TABLE 4.1   GENERAL

1	2	3	4
Colour	*Dress for Health*	*Psychological*	*Physiological*
MAGENTA	Royal and festive dress. In command but tacitly so. Only few can wear it often. Raising of energy level if not conscious enough.	Stimulating but lifting into richness of self, royal awareness. Self-respect. Dignity.	Individuality underlined. Composure
VIOLET	Peace and love involvement without anxiety. Concern, not worry. Authority without demand. Meditation and prayer. Good for balance and concentration.	Inner balance, reverence, silence, peacefulness. Individuality-enhancing.	Calming of body v. balance of mind. Sensuality raised.
BLUE	Quiet and settled, in control and, to the wearer, a relaxing dress. Lets others come near; lively person receives calm and offers peace.	Relaxing, unwinding, feeling of space.	Exhaling, relaxing of tension. Recharging energy to body.
TURQUOISE	A good support for people who are easily involved. Calming to nervous tensions. Non-dominating; fresh and young appearance.	Cooling, spacious, feeling fresh, new.	Pressure releasing Controlled exhaling towards release. Totally neutral, but good for objectivity.
GREEN	For those who are hyperactive, or need to be very active but wish not to be involved. Clear judgement. It offers no support but takes away no energy.	Arresting movement. Holding static. Balance. State of indecision.	Minimum liveliness. Held in place. Physical equilibrium. Can induce heat pulsations. Loss of memory.
YELLOW	Detachment from environment. Non-involvement. Good for those who wish to be alone and can be alone. Slightly unstabilising and insecure.	Detachment. Loss of reason and direction. Spacelessness. Loss of anchorage.	Shallow breathing. Irritable. Severing thought from action.
ORANGE	Joyful, and for people in need of joy. Anti-depressive, slightly detached and in a light mood. Not for those who need to be in authority.	Joy, lightness, release, pleasure, carefree attitude.	Ease in body. Relaxing of seriousness in thinking. Non-involvement. Sickly. Stifling.
RED	Lethargic person with lack of vitality, but well in health. Festive occasion. Need or want to be seen. Bad for those who tire easily. Commanding attention.	Stimulating, exciting, pleasurable. Alive, activating. Can be too much for some.	Inhaling. Inner tension to a degree of restriction, ending with exhaustion.

5	6	7	8	9	10
fect on Space	*Coloured Illumination on Matt Surfaces*	*Best Use in Decoration*	*Bad Use in Decoration*	*Supporting Form*	*Preferred Colour*
ace held in a mposed attitude. ontrolled feeling. ood concentra- on. Reassuring.	W. Peach blossom Y. Rose pink G. Blue B. De. blue R. De. orange Bl. De. violet	Chapels, entrance halls, lecture rooms	Entertainment areas	The cross; any strong vertical and horizontal shape	4.5%
hancing of ace, yet otected.	W. Lilac Y. L. pink G. L. slate B. Violet R. Da. orange Bl. Da. violet	Festive areas, grand-royal interior	Hospital wards, treatment rooms	Shelter, dome or tent effect; protection	6.5%
larging space. ne deeper the lour, the larger e space becomes.	W. L. blue Y. L. grey G. Turquoise B. De. blue R. De. purple Bl. Indigo	Bedrooms, office, treatment and stress areas	Not actively bad, dining and entertainment	Soft wave; calm horizontals	33%
ace free and esh, but still a lding effect.	W. L. green Y. P. green G. L. green B. Da. blue R. P. violet R. P. violet Bl. De. olive	Kitchens, bathrooms, some bedrooms and offices	Activity areas, playrooms.	Waves, clouds, peaks and reducing tall uprights	6.5%
ace made static. ead. Lethargic.	W. P. green Y. L. green G. Green B. Da. green R. Black Bl. Da. olive	Courtyards, external walls in towns, operating theatres	Most living and activity areas	Waves and horizontal planes	14.5%
ace lost. Taking way limitation. emoving nchorage.	W. Yellow Y. Yellow G. P. green B. Green R. L. red Bl. P. olive	Anti-depressive, light, mature mind environment	Offices, bedrooms, and work areas	Curves, loops and waves; movement	9.5%
ace balanced ut not restricted. ightly reducing.	W. De. yellow Y. De. orange G. Olive B. Slate R. P. red Bl. De. brown	Entertainment-dining area, passages	Bedrooms, studies, stress areas	Reducing starkness of space; creating buoyancy, loss of anchor	8.5%
educing space. ppressive when ense and strong.	W. Da. orange Y. P. red G. Black B. Black R. De. red Bl. Black	Entertainment and dancing	Bedrooms, offices, stress areas	All uprights: reducing height or increasing alertness	17%

KEY TO COLUMN 6

W. = white
Y. = yellow
G. = green
B. = blue
R. = red
Bl. = black

L. = light tone of colour ⎫   giving a gradual stepping down of shade seen
P. = pale tone of colour ⎬   under the eight illumination colours, i.e.
De. = deep tone of colour ⎬   magenta illumination on a white surface
Da. = dark tone of colour ⎭   produces peach blossom reflected colour

grew their hair, spoke in falsetto voices and sang soprano, metzo-soprano and alto. They looked and behaved like women. At the end of this whole period we had also become aware that their sex polarity had changed; emotionally they were now no longer men. Their beards grew less and less and their breast glands began to swell. I know it was not imagination, although *their* imaginations had started this development originally. The voice, or sounds which they used all the time now, had exercised their power over their bodies. A mantra sung, spoken or hummed regularly will induce a change, especially in a young human body.

The next ductless gland downward is the *heart*. This gland, as already described, has so much of the balancing energies within it. The colour associated with it is green and which points to the fact that we have in this centre of man a power of balance. It is said that the brain is an immature heart and that the heart, in a woman especially, is often used instead of the brain. (Brain energy can so easily be just a logical and intellectual output with which we can actually destroy our world.) The heart is the centre from which the balance and the love streams to preserve and protect.

Below the heart lies the *solar plexus*, associated with yellow. Its energies are the continuous flow of adjustment on the human level. Now that we come to the lower three glands we are also delving into the male colours. The glands below are the *adrenals*. These glands connect with the colour orange: the joy, the energy of renewal and, as medicine terms it, the genetic pattern.

Finally the *sacral gland* belongs with the colour red, the densest of all colours.

To gather up the element traces into the physical body so as to bring about maturity, it takes between twelve and sixteen years.

The division of the glandular system in the human being is a vast subject; the literature available is very diverse and offers to us many as yet unsolved questions. The comparison of one system with another, however, will widen the area of understanding. In this system we consider the heart as the central ductless gland. What is called a ductless gland in the medical profession may vary from the use of the term in this book. However, even among Doctors this term is undergoing changes. For the purpose of colour therapy we need to use the order described here.

Spirit, individuality	Magenta
Pineal/crown	Violet
Pituitary/third eye	Blue
Thyroid/throat	Turquoise
Cardiac plexus/heart	Green
Solar plexus/stomach	Yellow
Adrenals/side kidneys	Orange
Sacral/base	Red

After reflecting on this pattern, we must expand further on the complementary energy.

In the young person the red, orange and yellow colours dominate and come up from below to cover most of the field, the aura, around the body, whereas the blues and violets are narrow shafts coming down only gradually. These colours anchor and vitalise the child to become a member of the physical environment. We are now approaching the area which is known as the 'aura': the field of invisible energy around all physical beings, from humans to, and including, minerals. Even magnetism is a kind of aura. Colour plates 6(a), 6(b) and 6(c) show

how the aura changes in the course of maturing and from being in the denser colour realms (lower vibrations), the red spectrum gradually rises into the finer areas where the colour vibrations are less dense (faster vibrations) or the blue spectrum.

Part of growing up and becoming old is the joy of maturing and thereby being in a position of knowledge, wisdom, love and flexibility. This is made easier because the less dense colours enable the body to breathe in a wonderful way.

Auras, or Double Vibratory Vision

Very few people know that every child at the moment of birth has to reverse its perception. The upside-down world must become the right-way-up world and the colours must become the physical colours as we adults know them. This also holds good for the sound world. The form world in the child has completed this process at about eighteen months, or thereabouts, but the colour world takes a good deal longer, about six years. (Note here the 1 : 4 ratio of which rhythms there are so many found in human development.) Our whole system undergoes this change. As an embryo in the womb of the mother the only colour we *experience* is a deep blue. This colour is not even and dull, it is full of the radii and patterns of the veins, nerves and tissue density. It is subject also to changes of external light, day and night, and is affected further by electric light and the colours which are worn by the mother during pregnancy.

It may be good to keep to white, orange or red dress, as these colours do not interfere with the natural (reversed) colour perception of the embryo. After birth, this reversal of colours goes on for some time and, in some people, is never totally achieved. In these cases we have colour blindness.

Today people seek more and more to cope with awareness of their physical bodies. This coming to terms with physical matter as conscious people brings them closer and closer to the question: who are we? What is this matter of which we are made?

Light as we know it is obviously already a time element, but only a very little matter has here been absorbed. On a lower octave this is also experienced as sound.

Sound* has absorbed a good deal more density, therefore it is vibrating at an even lower level than light.** What is this vibration we call thought? During the investigation of such ideas we try to reach the purest state of thought possible by learning to set it apart from the body-bound experience. Such an activity we call meditation.

Meditation

Meditation is a way of using the human consciousness. It is based on the capacity to separate the two levels of being of man. The teachings handed down from antiquity are that man has the imprint of God and thus has the memory to be in communication with that part of his being. This being finds that by becoming visible it has separated itself from the ideal state of being. The art of communicating, even while in the physical body, depends on developing the capacity to leave this body, well protected like a locked house, and going on the return journey to find the origin.

This journey can be learned and it induces in the body a chemical, or equivalent to chemical, change which seems to produce the polarity effect to adrenalin, namely, a complete relaxation and almost death-like state. This can be observed in animals when in danger. Humans in that state find their consciousness then linked to a higher or broader level of awareness when in the ultimate state of this exercise. Time and space are removed and a vision can be obtained of what this being should do and how to conduct itself in this life in the physical body. Then problems arise which are the result of the free unattached spirit's attempt to translate the vision into the here and now. It is unwise to train young people with too little life experience and to open to them channels of communication which produce such problems as not to allow a continuation of everyday life because of the high level of frustration caused by the recognition that this vision cannot be put into effect in its ideal state. The

* Speed of sound = 1,100 feet per second. The vibrations audible to the human ear range between 30 and 22,000 cycles per second.
** $17 \cdot 5 \times 10^{15}$ = blue, $4 \cdot 6 \times 10^{14}$ = red. On either side of these vibrations ultra-violet and infra-red occur and there human vision can no longer see colour.

art is to come to terms with this, but to use the vision as a strength to aim for. More about this art will be found in Theo Gimbel: *Key, Lock and Door* (Hygeia Publications, Brook House, Avening, Gloucestershire, 1976). This is the gateway by which we start to extend our normal sight, our normal hearing, touch, taste and smell. Under usual circumstances, when we relax our bodies we go to sleep and are unconscious of the realms in which our minds travel. Using meditation in the correct way can help us to let our body go to sleep and our mind touch heightened vibrations. When we use meditation carefully and with good guidance, we begin to transcend our physical body and overcome the density little by little, in stages that bring about a chemical change in our bodies. Slowly we raise our vibrations and become aware of this timeless communication with people and places. We could then say that we begin to lift our normal sight into the next octave above, when we become aware of the less dense vibrations. We cannot say actually that we 'see' as such; but that we 'perceive' or 'experience'. We begin to live in the vibrations of our environment.

Those who develop such gifts must also develop a moral responsibility towards their use. Never must they be used for the wrong reasons. There are two kinds of double vibratory rate: (a) that naturally available from birth and (b) that later achieved by training and through work. Those who have been endowed with this gift of clairvoyance can be said to fall into two particular groups: one in which it is unwise to give any teaching by those of us who have trained to achieve this stage of perfection; and the other group to whom it may be advisable to give help and training which brings about increased and more selective use of this gift.

Those who have learnt this will usually, when well trained, know that they have the choice of using the gift or not, according to the circumstance in which they find themselves. When a high degree of morality has been developed along with this double-vibratory vision, then the restricted use will not be so necessary as it is at the beginning. All circumstances in which it is used should involve the healing help we offer to our fellow beings and environment. By this is meant earth, plant, animal and man, as these are all interdependent. Sickness and disease follow where the density for each of these kingdoms becomes too great, when in each the held density brings about a state of static being, which takes that particular animal, plant or man out of the necessary flow and the changes which are important for this being to be well.

Aura Forms

How do we begin to know the measure of change, the flow and the forms which prevail around, and as a result of, their various levels of density? Let us being with the minerals. In them we experience a very fast inflow of vibrations, the degree of which tells us about the density level. The faster the inflow, the denser the matter. As an answer to this inflow there is a counter-outflow of vibrations. In minerals these outflowing energies are so slow that we men cannot usually perceive them.

STONE

As a start, in training, one can use a small stone and hold it in the palm of one's hand. After some time the holder will begin to feel the counter-vibration which, in this case, is his own pulse beat throbbing against the stone. Then we can say after all that this stone is alive, in so far as it can give us a measure of self-awareness. We may have regarded it as dead because we have had to start with no perception, not even conceptions with which to measure the life of that stone. Now we begin to realise that we do find a life in it, albeit so slow that we can only stand in awe of this deep level of being. IT HAS TAKEN UP DENSITY SO THAT WE MAY BE SPARED THIS. At this stage I would like to say that the opening words of the Bible *can* be understood as follows: 'IN THE BEGINNING GOD *BECAME* HEAVEN AND EARTH . . .' Thus we hold some part of God in our hands when we hold a stone. This vibration is the foundation on which we stand. One day, through our own thinking, it must return to those highest vibrations beyond what we in the physical form call light. This view of the mineral world is not a common one, but is recommended that it is referred to again later, when some of the following content adds further understanding.

PLANT

Now we take into our perception a plant; the inflowing vibrations are slower than those of the mineral kingdom, but the counter-flow is more perceptible as it is raised to a faster outflow than that of the stone. (By the rates of these outflowing vibrations the clairvoyant can estimate the usefulness of the help that both these kingdoms can offer to man in easing his disease.)

Plants have much to offer man as there is a great affinity between us and them. Again, because of this affinity, man, the mediator between the two (the plant and the invisible), is given the gift of freedom from density. Plants receive man's attitudes and can respond to what a human being is thinking and feeling; they also grow by this as much as by his actions.

ANIMAL

The animal world has descended entirely into the physical plane. In their various forms animals have taken up many of the restrictions which, by their acceptance of them, man is spared. Their inflow light, or aura colours, are slow and their outflow patterns are fast. Speed again varies between reptile, mammal or bird. Reptiles draw in faster than birds and let go more slowly. Mammals take up a kind of middle position. These creatures have, in their density and limitation, made it possible for man to achieve more freedom and adaptability. Because of their limitations, they are more filled with fear and aggression towards all that approaches them in an atmosphere of fear. However, the many meeting which have been experienced between animals and man always point out that these creatures below us can help with all their varied specialised energies. Not only do fairy tales tell of the connections of animal and man, of a wonderful co-operation; but also there are present-day experiences which confirm this as reality.

Here is a story which illustrates well the sort of response a big Italian sheepdog showed to me. I was warned not to rise from my place and was left alone with the beautiful creature lying by the table, watching me all the time. Her owner said: 'Stay in your seat and she is perfectly all right.' A moment after my host had left, I got up as I wanted to go to my car to fetch a book. The sheepdog, wild and growling, with open mouth, came towards me and grabbed my left hand ready to tear out some skin and flesh. How one thinks so fast I do not know, but faced with the apparently inevitable, I instantly put the dog and myself into an orb of light and love. The dog at once let go of my hand and licked it all over, pressing her beautiful large body against my side. Such are the aura reflec- tions at such a moment and all this seems to be read by animals and acted upon without hesitation. We men can sometimes do this, but we have to overcome our blocks to a large extent.

HUMAN

By and large an aura is like an egg. It has both horizontal and vertical energy patterns. The vertical ones ray out and in, whilst the horizontal ones breathe, pulsating sometimes gently, some- times very fast. This movement depends upon the activity which is taking place at any moment in the mind, soul and body of that person. As a result of the slightest change, either voluntary or involuntary, the aura patterns dance and vibrate, change colour to some extent and reflect all that goes on in the person. Past, present and future are also there but one must have a great deal of experience before one uses the double vibratory vision for diagnosis. Those who have had a lot of experience become great helpers in the visible world. Finally, one must also take into account that every clairvoyant has developed his or her own individual method in this field and accounts do differ, but diagnosis will always be correct provided the necessary experience is there and discipline has been observed.

The experience of aura reading is like a question and answer that takes place at a speed which is akin to the double vibratory vision, only it is in the sound area instead. Translating this into human language often causes difficulty, but there again, with more and more work in this field one can gain better translation in time.

Drug-Taking

Individual aura patterns differ enormously. Here I should like to quote three particular cases of drug-taking and the effect it can have on the aura. Let us take Figure 4.3(a) as the normal pattern of the etheric sheath and relate the following three cases to this.

(1) In this case (Figure 4.3b) there are, at almost regular intervals, vertical wedges of black driven from outside into the centre. These have started to drive themselves into the etheric layer at about 3–4½in from the physical body. This is a highly dangerous stage and will be very hard to put right. The remainder of the aura is weak and all colours have a greyish tint. It would be recommended that this person should not only eat, drink and be in the environment of healthy natural things, but

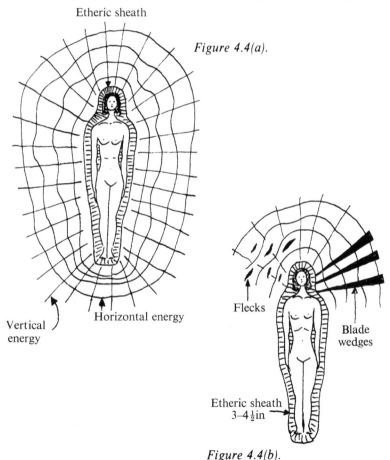

Etheric sheath

Figure 4.4(a).

Vertical energy

Horizontal energy

Flecks

Blade wedges

Etheric sheath 3–4½in

Figure 4.4(b).

also accompany rest periods and going to sleep with the conscious use of 'exchange breathing' recommended for clearing your body from density and rejuvenating the body, soul and spirit. (See Theo Gimbel: *Key, Lock and Door* Hygeia Publications, 1973; chapter on exchange breathing.)

(2) The aura has faded away to a very light green (Figure 4.4c); which is not a good aura colour at the best of times. Green is not a natural human aura colour and when it is present it can indicate a dangerous state of weakness in the body of the person concerned. Again it is recommended to have as much natural intake as possible of food and air and conscious exchange

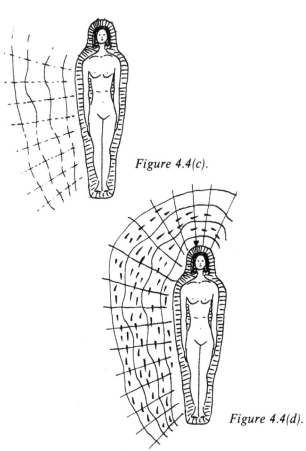

Figure 4.4(c).

Figure 4.4(d).

breathing is vital. Such persons have to rescue themselves by building their aura again very deliberately. A great deal of teaching is necessary so that they can do this properly.

(3) This produces a most beautiful aura, with very clear colours, predominantly light violet-rose, and excellent patterns, both vertical and horizontal. However (Figure 4.4d), light grey-blue flecks in the horizontal patterns indicate that the person has smoked 'grass' – just one cigarette already shows. Such flecks can be dissolved very easily at comparatively little cost to health.

Human Communication with Other Kingdoms

The centre in which man places himself, namely, his body, is capable of reaching out into the universe as well as being subdued by the energies of intensity of light and sound. High wattage electric light used in conjunction with colour and sound pushed through amplifiers make the 'centre' feel dominated and manipulated into the depths of subconsciousness. Technology, harnessing the mineral elements through the knowledge of inter-reaction, dulls down the human consciousness. We need only to be subjected to flashing lights and amplified sound to know that there is no peace, no contemplation, no actual consciousness possible; under such conditions man is driven into a graceless ugly shape, jerking and twitching to the lights and sounds. A person who subjects his body to these influences causes his being to be densified into the three colours which lie below the green balance of the heart.

On the other hand, a human being who can calm the body to the state of consciousness of an animal, which produces predominantly alpha rhythms, can communicate with this kingdom very significantly. By further careful relaxing of this body we reach into the realm in which Father Andrew Glazewski was such a master. Communication with plants and trees is only ultimately possible if we let our body relax further and the central nervous system tunes into ceta waves. The high sensitivity level of plants is just now in the process of being discovered by such people as Marcel Vogel and Cleve Backster. We delve now into the realm where we communicate with plants in their own rhythms. However, man should not attempt to do this unless he is sure how to handle the realm of this consciousness. Finally, and only at present through highly developed mastery of the human body by mind control, we can tune into the state of delta waves in which the whole mineral world is vibrating. Again, the person doing this needs to know how to return safely into the state of beta after having tapped such high atunement.

The colours which man reaches are, in this case, of the order of indigo, lifting himself out of this into gold, then into magenta. In this order we can say:

animals	— alpha	= indigo
plants	— ceta	= gold
minerals	— delta	= magenta

Interestingly, after reaching such a state, but only very rarely, we tap the realm beyond, which is beauty: a significant timeless and spaceless experience of the divine realm of angels – God's realm.

The state described earlier in this chapter under the heading 'meditation' is also known as the reuniting with the angels which are in charge of the energies when all their complete, complex and awe-inspiring world is approached, when the incomprehensible, ever-expanding being becomes God as understood by all humans in all religions.

Visions of Angels

Michelangelo had a vision when he painted the famous Madonna. The background of his painting depicts innumerable angels filling all the heavens beyond. The vision must have been an unforgettable experience for this great artist. May I offer an experience which to me is equally unforgettable and contained the teaching which gave me the above concept of the state of an angel. While I was dressing one morning, suddenly the whole room seemed to be full of angels. Rapidly their presence filled the garden, the landscape beyond, indeed all the universe was a complete sea of these beings. At the same time I was 'told': You are seeing the edge of the little finger of God. Simultaneously I seemed to understand that every cell is an energy, hence there is an angel hidden behind the cell of all that is visible here and now.

To reach the state of complete relaxation and total peace is life-preserving – the best chance of surviving in a crisis situation. This is very well described in Lyall Watson's book *The Romeo Error* Hodder and Stoughton 1974. It is experienced in the finest distribution of magenta, mostly not recognised as colour but as a brilliant, but not dazzling, pure light. The inner colours as described above are graduating towards more and more light. This light is not, however, the light which we see around us with our eyes but the light which we can call the inner light that exists in the darkness. Blind people can describe this state very well. This magenta, so finely present, is the highest energy which we can perceive at this present stage of evolution, being in the physical body. Thereby our vision of God is limited, but not blocked. The already-mentioned scale of density (see Figure 4.3) is once more brought to our mind and we can see now how much the balance 'colour' plays in this scale.

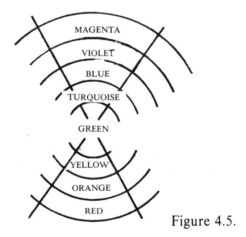

Figure 4.5.

Darkness and Light in Healing

When human beings need healing it must be understood that darkness plays an enormous part in that process. Good sleep is available through darkness. When light is needed it should be a blue light that gently draws the mind into the healing distance in which we can relax and shed such density as we have wrongly accumulated. Blue helps us to expand, relax and sleep. The light which then shines into this darkness is like the primaeval mother (darkness) being greeted by the primaeval father (light). Between these two great beings arises the third being (colour).

Colour appears always at the edge between the visible and invisible world, the manifested and the non-manifested. We can actually touch the subtle parts of nature which are either on the way to becoming visible, or to becoming invisible again.

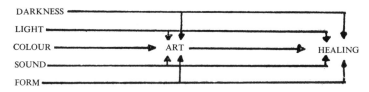

Degrees of density and their use in art and healing.

When the two lightest edges of the natural spectrum overlap the colour green appears. This mysterious colour holds an amazing balance. Nature, or at least the plant world, is predominantly green. There are dozens of different shades of green: one can take real pleasure in looking at a mixed border of plants before these have started to flower. What does green do to our psyche? What do we actually experience when we are in a green environment? To me it is always a wonderful sensation as the greens in nature play upon my whole being and finely stimulate my feeling of balance. No more and no less than that. I am, in fact, held in balance by this colour; not, however, in a dead balance but in that intangible, hovering, gently swaying middle that does not produce the static immobility which occurs when green is used as pigment and a room is painted with a flat green paint. (See Appendix I, 'Growing Plants Under Colour'.) In green we meet the optical adjustment of the retina and focus neither behind nor in front of the retina, but actually on the retina.

The Spectrum

When we bring together the two deepest ends of the spectrum (pages 84 and 93) – violet and red – we come to a colour which is the polarity of green. We call this magenta. This colour seems to rise out of the darkness and offers us a most astonishing impression. We are lifted out of the darkness and experience the colour that is set opposite the green. Magenta holds the result of the whole spectrum. Finely distributed, it is the peach blossom colour, the colour of man.

Colours impress us most in our younger years. The rainbow is the most obvious natural phenomenon where pure colours are seen. It appears opposite the source of light against a darker background when the atmosphere is saturated with moisture. It is a perfect arc (part of a circle). It is the breaking of light through a fine body of density, water or glass.

When we take colours in isolation, e.g. blue, and produce an even spread of this without the natural fade into turquoise or indigo, then we are holding in a static position one particular, immeasurably fine part of the spectrum. To some extent we have taken it like a fish out of water which soon must either die or be related back into its element of completeness.

Colours used as decor differ from colours used as light (shining through a filter). These two are in some respects complementary. To a very fine degree two different blues, however small the difference may be, create between them a sort of spectrum completion. This is true for all colours. Any colour used as pigment and decoration works quite deliberately. As we perceive its visual image we can always remind ourselves of this colour 'blue'. Thus the impact of this colour is made via our sense perceptions. We can at any moment remind ourselves of the colour and say that it is blue. Nevertheless, it also has a subconscious impact which is quite significant; for example, while getting used to a decoration colour we do not often remind ourselves of the colour consciously (Rudolf Steiner, '*Spritual Science and Medicine*' Rudolf Steiner Press, London, 1975).

When we examine colour in detail, (see plate 7 between pages 84 and 93) we see that there are eight main colours; these are subdivided again by a further eight, such as the range green/yellow to orange/yellow, with a whole octave within

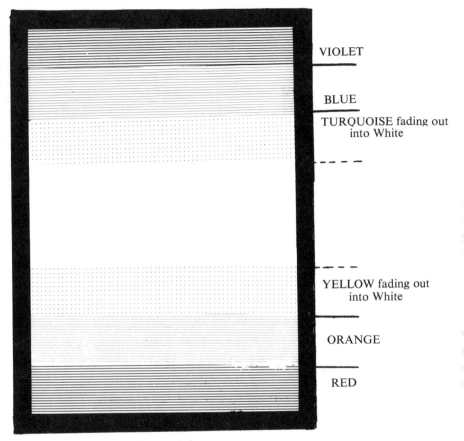

VIOLET

BLUE

TURQUOISE fading out
into White

YELLOW fading out
into White

ORANGE

RED

Figure 4.6.

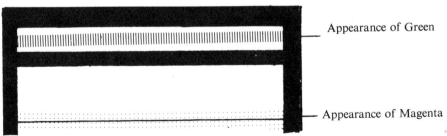

Appearance of Green

Appearance of Magenta

Figure 4.7.

yellow. When illuminating a room this plays an important part and a living or a dead light can appear according to the choice we make. Light is not just a thing that makes some dark place visible but, like darkness, it has a body with which it can fill a space. According to the source, it can be beneficial or detrimental to human health.

Using not only an ordinary tungsten bulb but combining it with coloured filters we can arrange a most beautiful light which, though not as perfect as daylight, is far more beneficial than the ordinary 100-watt frosted bulb. From long research and experience we know that wall-mounted lights are better than ceiling-suspended. These can be shaded off with gentle colours and adjusted accordingly by way of transistorised switches. For example of how to use colour and environment see Table 4.1 on page 51.

Use of Colour in Decor

Red rooms and illumination are invigorating, producing activity, but if totally so decorated and illuminated they will induce violence, which produces an imbalance of the human mental activity by conduction through the nerves as described earlier. Football is often watched under strong illumination. If sodium vapour lamps are used they have a high red level and are manipulative to a fairly high degree. It may be that cricket is watched in daylight (which has an enormously high blue content) it is, therefore, not conducive to violence. The calming down of a violent crowd was achieved by Gerrard and Hessey in 1932, by using blue illumination.

Red-orange coloured patterns are compelling. The more complex the pattern, the more absorbing will it be to the person facing it. Here is some good business advice on how to be in command of, even if manipulating your customer. A bank manager's room is painted deep blue on three walls; the wall behind his desk is decorated with a high class red-orange, very complex wallpaper design. The customer cannot take his mind or interest away from it. Some time later he finally had worked out the repeat pattern, which is very well hidden. The voice of the bank manager comes back to him saying, 'Now all you have to do is sign here ...' 'But what on earth is it all about?' goes through the customer's mind. He has not taken in what has been said, and will not expose the fact by asking for it to be repeated. The customer is taken unawares and not in control.

Blue rooms and illumination make for a calming, expanding, relaxing environment with much more space (red decreases space) to sleep in; also they can minimise anxiety in waiting rooms in hospitals, doctors' consulting rooms or antenatal clinics.

Turquoise is more calming to nervous dispositions and is suitable for hospitals, or for the study of an overtaxed, strained company director.

Blue-violet is a warm blue, comforting, good for those who suffer from claustrophobia and asthma and a state of inferiority complex which this colour can help to reduce.

Violet: dignified, devout, religious or pious; such are the psychic influences on those who are in a violet room with violet illumination.

Magenta enhances the effect of violet with a desire to be lifted out of the involvement of our present demanding world, avoiding challenges; it can be too relaxing, ultimately dangerous to those who have a tendency to opt out, and may induce suicide out of pure desire not to be burdened any longer. On the other hand, however, it could be used for a space in a terminal ward, where people wish, to die in a dignified environment.

Yellow decor and illumination as a complete scheme is not congenial to our present state. It is a fallacy to think 'nice and bright'. Using this colour exclusively, we quickly reach a state of mind where the anchors which the multi-coloured environment offers to us have been removed.

Green decoration and illumination will place the person into a static environment. It will not promote vitality, not does it assist relaxation. It can become a tiring experience as the occupant of the room has to do both relaxing and being active without the help of the colour. The illumination (green) is of all the colours the most unpleasant and can deplete very quickly. It can be said to have a cleansing effect, but that, like fasting, is a time at which a person should physically not be active; in this case he may almost be rendered incapable!

GENERAL REMARKS:
It is not easy for anyone to be objective and balanced when making a choice of colours for one's own use. Subconsciously or superconsciously, we may always choose the right environment. To come concretely to a decision means to detach oneself first and move out of the way of one's own problems. Hence a colour therapist has a job to do. It is still as well to remember, however, that even the therapist has in the training been instructed how to remove his or her personal problems or blocks before a patient is being counselled or taken into a colour therapy session.

The Language of Colours

This appraisal of the use of colours for stage lighting is based on the studies which Max Gümbel-Seiling (my father) made from work done with Rudolf Steiner in München between the years 1912 and 1925.

Generally, use:

Light colours for young or inexperienced, innocent persons
Saturated colours for impressive personalities
Gold for personalities endowed with wisdom

It must be remembered that my father had great insight into anthroposophy and that some of the meanings he has used in the above are taking it for granted that the reader is familiar with Steiner's work. However, some of the general ideas will become clearer when the lighting for a play is set up using his advice; and the experience will then show the way to further, and indeed enlarge, the above in the light of modern thinking.

The Hue	*Atmosphere*	*Quality*	*Effect*
	(Rainbow)	Spiritual	
WHITE	Beyond the realm of the soul	The soul's picture of the spirit	Festive and joyful

The Hue	Atmosphere	Quality	Effect
BLACK	Silence	Spiritual image of death	Gruesome (fear)
GREY	Undecided	Dawn/dusk	Fearsome (uneasy)
RED	Stimulating to action and for wonder, awe	Shine of the living	Joyfully active
ORANGE	Personal warmth of soul, insufficiency and preferences		Stimulating
YELLOW	In nature inwardly stabilised	Radiating	Inner liveliness
GREEN	The gate for wonder	Dead image of life	
BLUE	Sympathy and antipathy about all development	Raying inwards	(Passive)
INDIGO	Overflowing soul		
VIOLET	Border of the supersensible desire to pray		Festive, sincere
MAGENTA/ PEACH BLOSSOM		Living picture of the soul	Transition into the spiritual

The Hue	*Soul of Colour*	*Desire Aspect*	*Practical Use*
BROWN			Dry, matter-of-fact
	(Life of the individuality)	Effect of the body on the soul	
WHITE	Shining	Hazy (blunt), message from above x	Angel, bride, supersensible person
BLACK	To appear invisible	Threat from below x	Devil, priest, judge
GREY	Warning	Lackadaisical	Ghost, boarder towards below x
RED	Pink: loving, contended, the joy of activity	Pink: selfless natural instinct, fury, lust, pleasure	
ORANGE	Self-opinionated, inquisitive	Ambition, pride	
YELLOW	Bright, Intelligent, clear-thinking	Amber: passion	Intelligent, important, clever persons
GREEN	Understanding of the world and life	Dim-witted and lazy, comfortable	
BLUE	Devotion, piety	Good-tempered, removed from the world	Melancholy

The Hue	*Soul of Colour*	*Desire Aspect*	*Practical Use*
INDIGO	Idealism		Sincere
VIOLET	Religious devotion	Magic, compelling, spell	Mystical, very old, border towards the above x
MAGENTA/ PEACH BLOSSOM	Desire to dematerialise	Determined to the soul aspect	
BROWN	Tendency to become fixed	Earth-bound, intimate	Earth-bound souls

Order and Significance of the Eight Colours

Let us now consider the eight colours as they occur in the spectrum.

RED is the colour which is used to attract the conscious mind when it is applied in decor or for a poster. However, it also rejects penetration, or any prolonged viewing. Psychologically a little goes a long way, in either time or space. In any surroundings it is the colour which is first noticed by the visual perception. Rooms decorated in red appear smaller than they are. A ceiling can be lowered by red, but it has an unpleasant psychological impact upon people, a feeling of oppression and weight from above. It can cause claustrophobia where otherwise such a condition would not appear. Only a few people need it as a constant environment in the northern hemisphere. Within us it creates the feeling of excitement, stimulation and warmth.

The social structure of law by intellect, the complexity of daily life with all its technology, from childhood to the end of life, being on the look-out for accident-prone situations involving traffic, etc., the pressure of existence because of the drive towards improved living standards, even education, being a competitive business, all creates an anxiety level which has the same effect as being in a red environment.

Turquoise is the complementary colour.

Decoration A red room is where activity takes place. To stimulate a monotonous action can be the outcome of a red workshop where people quickly tire of doing the same thing for hours. Red is also suitable for a room in which we wish to be alert and experience our activity on a higher level of excitement. To celebrate festivities and for amusement, red is a good decoration colour.

Light Like blue light, red light is powerful and leads to the raising of the pulse beat; inhalation is stimulated and consciousness is collected. Self-awareness increases and one achieves an alert state which raises consciousness and facilitates judgement of mental attitudes.

Witty remarks and teasing are encouraged; but again, the slightly varied red decoration with red illumination brings about a spectrum effect that is much more powerful than just one single usage of red. In a varied environment we are extended and externalised; hence exposure- and movement-activating forces are dominating.

When sluggishness and lack of stimulus is experienced, when all action is an effort beyond the normal, when there is no physiological reason why this state should prevail, it is a help to be exposed to a concentration of red-green/blue-red rhythm. Paralysis is also beneficially influenced by this colour. When using any colour care should be taken, but especially so with red.

ORANGE contains both yellow and red. It is a joyful colour, protected from both the overstimulation of red and the detaching effect of yellow. Dining-room areas, kitchens and playrooms benefit from this colour.

Blue is the complementary colour. (Orange and blue tones make for a very successful interior when used with care and discretion.)

Decoration Best used in rooms for young people.

Light Still stimulating and movement enhancing.

In many cases orange can be used to enliven an otherwise lethargic attitude or condition. As light, it influences the whole of the human system strongly, but not as vigorously as red.

YELLOW is the colour nearest to light. This colour is needed by all living beings. Yellow light, when used as a contrast to a natural setting where blue is dominant and other colours sup-

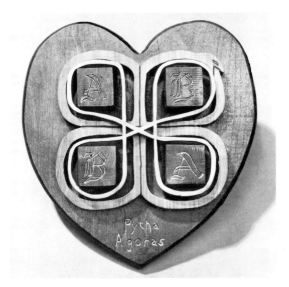

Plate 1 The Seal of Pythagoras *(see page 47)*

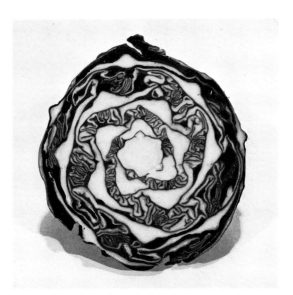

Plate 2 Here we see a red cabbage cut in such a way as to reveal three spirals which make up a network of energy lines. Between each rib it is possible to draw the interconnecting ones and thus find a pentagram inscribed into the organic development of the plant *(see page* 84.)

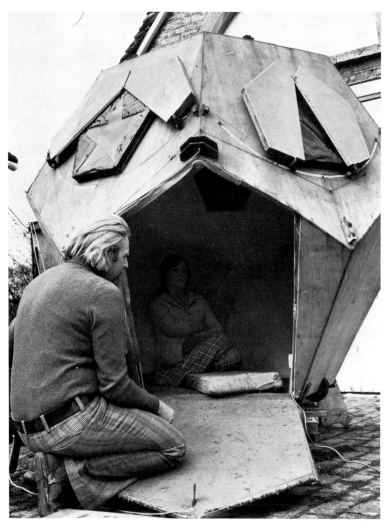

Plate 3 A working model of the colour therapy room *(see page 121)*

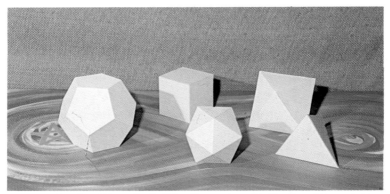

Plate 4 The five Platonic Solids: Ether, Earth, Water, Air and Fire *(see page 29)*

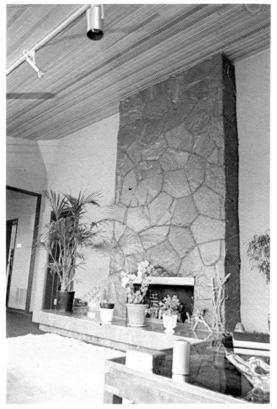

Plate 5 The Triangular Conversion *(see page 123)*

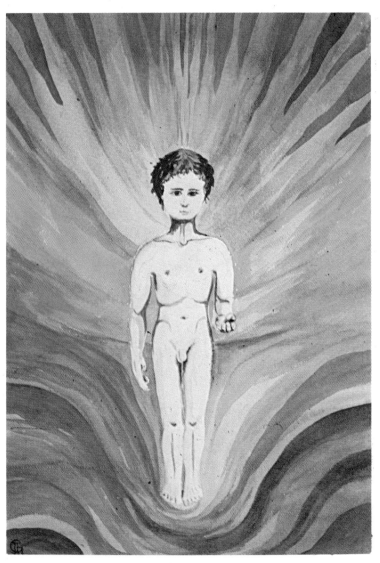

Plate 6 (a) the young aura

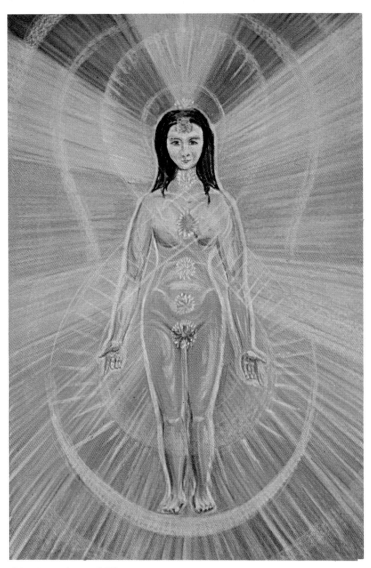

(b) the prime of life aura

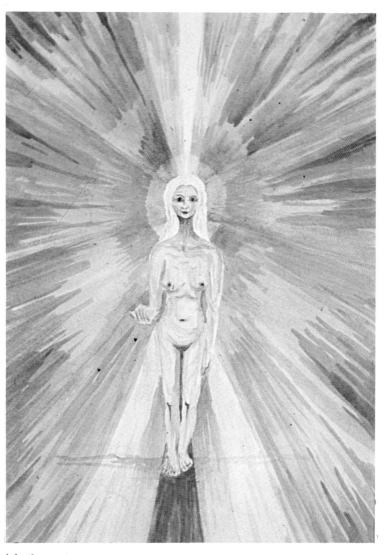

(c) the mature aura

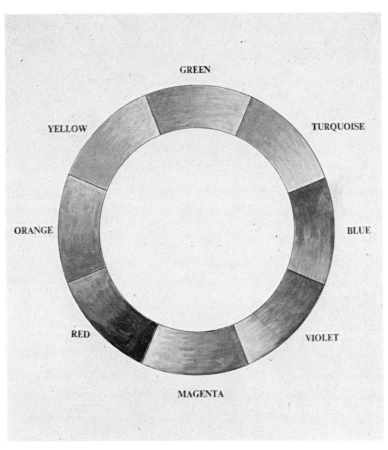

Plate 7 The Spectrum of the Eight Colours *(see page* 77*)*

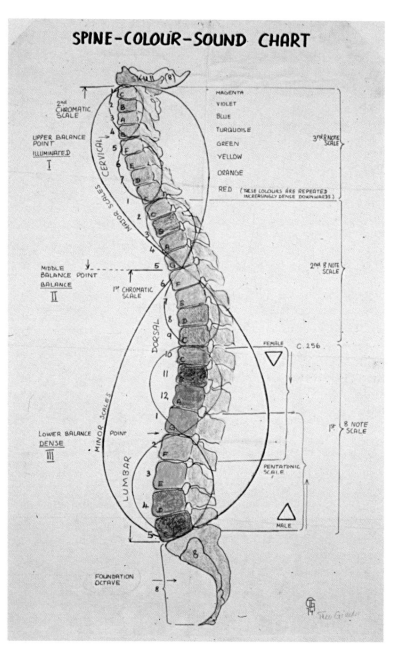

SPINE-COLOUR-SOUND CHART

Plate 8 *(see page 110)*

port, is the light to elevate the human psyche and spirit. In the environment it is available as daylight and enhanced or exaggerated by electric light at night. The colour is more delicate than either of the other two primary colours. It is very quickly changed from a pure yellow into green or orange. As it is a colour which has to do with direction, moving from centre to periphery, or as a beam sending out its rays into a selected area, it is not a colour that stands easily by itself. The use of it in a pure unadulterated form is inadvisable as its mental impact is a loss of anchorage or protection, aim or focus. Several accounts are available to show that yellow light combined with yellow decoration is not a good environment for humans. A detachment from consciously responsible behaviour quickly sets in and people act irrationally. Nervousness is encouraged and uncertainty appears. Even violence has been sparked off by yellow light, especially if the person subjected to this colour has not a firm plan of action in mind.

Violet is the complementary colour.

Decoration It is inadvisable as the only colour in any room. Neither shelter nor direct stimulation can be experienced.

Light The illumination of a room with yellow has an uplifting effect, provided the room contains plenty of everyday objects with a good balance of colour from the rest of the spectrum. Using a yellow room and yellow light together should be guarded against – the effect may be disastrous. Yellow light can be beneficial in cases of arrested movement. Again, it is of vital importance that it is carefully applied and measures are taken to ensure that, in cases of arthritis, there are no other reasons for the stiffness or loss of movement, such as paralysis (see red).

GREEN When light has penetrated into water or earth the green life of the plant kingdom rises, and yet the green is transformed light which has 'died' into matter; thus green has been described as the 'dead image of life'. Once something has become green, the next step is decay. The special place green has in the spectrum points to the fact that it holds special powers. (See Appendix I, 'Growing Plants Under Colour'.)

Magenta is the complementary colour.

Decoration For reasons of its unlimited shades in nature, its ever-changing hues, green used as a decoration in a room is rarely a success. It becomes dead, flat and empty. Our eyes and

93

the whole of our body feel deprived and impoverished when green is used as a flat paint.

Light   Green light is never pleasant: it reminds us of past life, of something that was once alive. Used in colour-light work it prevents the growth and further adding of matter in living organisms. Green decoration with green lighting is a very strong environment to use in design. Unless growth has gone out of order they should not be used together and, if used, they must be very carefully guided and watched in their effects.

TURQUOISE is a cool, refreshing colour with a morning appearance, calming and soothing, especially when heat and pressure have been endured.

Red is the complementary colour.

Decoration   This is somewhat more successful in interior decoration than green. The area becomes larger but still holds a sufficiency of static appearance.

Light   Cool and detached. Not advisable for living, play or work. Illumination will be applied to 'cool down' temperature and nervous inflammations.

BLUE is the colour which is predominant today throughout the world. Blue is needed by the majority of human beings. It creates within us a feeling of calm and taking the hurry and bustle out of life; a relaxation from the stimulating environment to which most people are constantly exposed. More and more we are surrounded with exciting colour, startling posters, and colour is crammed on to a surface that is too small to hold the amount. Scientifically speaking, the phosphorus colour pigments are using a method that I would call the misuse of chemistry. It produces a shouting, almost unavoidable density of colour, which can become practically unbearable to sensitive people.

Orange is the complementary colour to blue.

Decoration   When people are subjected to a blue room (walls decorated with blue paint), a feeling of breathing out results. Blue objects appear larger than they really are. An excited person is calmed, breathing is slowed down and exhaling is encouraged. The room might, perhaps, be called cool, but this is not really so. There are warm blues and cool blues, as much as there are cool reds and warm reds.

Light   A much-enhanced calming effect can be obtained from blue light. We may have noticed the impact of the blue at the beginning when we entered the room, but very soon we become accustomed to it and lose the physical sense of coloured light. Blue light in a blue room (decor) has a very powerful effect; the pulse is lowered and the exhaling is deeper; a feeling of release and retreat into a shelter is the overall result.

Thus blue can be used to help in all those cases where the tensions and restrictions of the ordinary environment have produced a state of ill health. Asthmatic conditions can be helped considerably by blue as a colour (decor) and used as a light. The reinforcement of blue is at times very desirable and it can be produced by using the complementary colour, or even red.

An individual rhythm between the amount of blue and the red must be found for each person. This can only be done by experience and the proper usage of instruments. It is, therefore, most important to have a training and a full understanding of the whole nature of colour and man before the right rhythms can be found. It has also been very significant in allowing the person who wishes to have such help to express fully, through all his faculties, his own nature. Out of this and with the help of consultants who have insight into this field, one will arrive at the right sequence, rhythms, time and intensity of a beneficial colour-light application.

VIOLET   This colour is related to the human mentality. Composed as it is of blue and red it bears within it on the one hand the shelter, capacity of embrace, relaxing, and on the other the stimulant, rousing into activity which is inherent in red. What do we get when those two activities are joined? Submission to the other space which embraces us and the concentration directed towards a specific purpose. Another word for it is prayer or meditation.

The colour has such a balancing effect that we are offered an environment in which we are balanced in a way as with green, yet on a completely different level. The actual places for healing, however, are better in blue, or turquoise, depending on the need of the patient. This change is easily made by having a mobile illumination source such as a colour-level lamp.

Yellow is the complementary colour.

Decoration   Areas where dignity is necessary, entrance halls for hospitals, places of worship and dedication.

Light   Violet illumination creates peace and tranquillity; on wood of honey-coloured shades it produces almost a gold sheen. It is the light of blessing and remembrance of a higher potential. Used as a light source it has a gentle contracting effect, often for inflammations which are still not clear from an infection and will not draw together and be expelled from the body.

MAGENTA   Like green, this colour is not available naturally unless we bring about a physical condition by which the red and the violet begin to mix. It is a very spiritual colour which has a humanising effect. When, through the pressure of daily life, we are irate or worried, out of tune and feel inwardly savage and angry, the colour draws us out of this non-human attitude. Magenta completes the spectrum as it is the octave (eighth) colour which we use in connection with this work. It is a kind of fulfilment colour. When one feels contentment, having achieved a balance between the psychic and the emotional and mental state, this colour induces a beautiful feeling of completeness.

Decoration   It will not be easy to produce a pure shining magenta as in the colour-mixing violet and red will not easily yield a clean hue. This colour is very elusive and easily slides into hues which are no longer magenta. It is advisable to use a prism.

Light   Magenta light is uplifting into a realm which stands beyond the physical, an experience which leads closely to the spiritual.

The light is sobering and deep in its impact upon the mentality of man. Together with a violet decor it would act as a primaeval and futuristic death and re-birth situation; it should therefore not be used unless very careful preparations have been made and every aspect of the circumstances points to the advisability of using it. Of all the combinations, this is the most powerful one, holding past and future, and by placing the present situation into this frame we will extend into experiences that have deep healing possibilities. It can be said that it had such a high quality of healing power that the use of it might well be described as an experience of excarnation: when the spirit frees itself from the physical. In very rare cases it might help to clear away accumulated darkness which has distorted the thoughts and choked the filters which give man access to the realm of the spiritual world. Excarnation is another term for death but means in its fuller sense the the life is continued on a non-physical level. Some of the great adepts have 'excarnated' themselves, meaning that they were able to dissolve their physical bodies and return to the spirit state.

BLACK is the extreme, the visible world going over into the invisible, the spiritual. In this outer darkness there rises the light, the inner of the spirit. The dark end touches the point of night, the holy darkness. All experiences are attached to black. It is lucid, more transparent, easily accessible to both positive and negative impact. In the colour scale it stands at the end of red and the beginning of violet. Magenta rises out of it as a phoenix from the dead.

WHITE All is excluded from it. White is purity in itself as a non-experience. Both black and white hold the total potentially within them.

White is the ultimate purity, the untouched, the innocence of all beings. It used to be the priests' colour and in some orders still is. But it has, as the other hand, isolation and all is excluded from it. A completely white space is as terrifying as totally black environment.

BROWN is the colour of integration and offering, even sacrifice. The autumn leaves in nature commit the life energy of the sun to the earth in their 'death' process. As a colour it is also found in rust, which is often very close to orange. Iron ore, when pure and clean, is almost the complementary colour to rust: a deep indigo greyish blue. Brown as a colour in many polished woods shows this final attempt the plants have made to integrate into this world.

GREY is the colour of denial, perhaps of all the colours the most negative, the colour of self-denial and evasion, non-commitment, and in its worst role the weakness of a lie, the result of complete destruction in ashes. In spite of this it can show off all the other bright colours, in exhibitions, etc., without taking anything away.

Red ⎫
Yellow ⎭ Orange ⎫
⎬ BROWN
Red ⎫ ⎪
Blue ⎭ Violet ⎭

Mixing these primary colours thus we obtain brown. It is also the colour of steel when allowed to rust. Compare the indigo steel blue and the rust colour: there are the complementary forces at play again.

Blue ⎫
Yellow ⎭ Green ⎤
　　　　　　　⎬ SLATE
Blue ⎫　　　 ⎪
Red ⎭ Violet ⎦

Slate or grey is not a colour which is comfortable; it is the colour of shyness, indecision, uncertainty. The overtones of this colour make for a kind of escape from clarity and pleasure. Depression is often grey and lacks strength.

Yellow ⎫
Blue ⎭ Green ⎤
　　　　　　　⎬ OLIVE
Yellow ⎫　　 ⎪
Red ⎭ Orange ⎦

A colour which has deep maturity, almost indicating decay, on the verge of death. It is nondescript, unassertive, a negation of life and joy, also in some ways depressive.

All these three colours can be used to offset other colours and make them more effective. When used sparingly and intelligently, many fine results in interior decoration can be achieved.

The designer will find by experimentation in each individual case many combinations where, in an otherwise red room, grey can be used to give the background for some special picture or ornament. Slate, as mentioned above, tends to the blue. Conversely, in a blue room, the lightish brown, with a tendency to orange, is very agreeable. Olive used in an orange to yellow room serves as grey can for red.

The illumination levels which we use are not always the best degree of either brilliance or restraint. Also, they often lack a particular tone which could have been more beneficial. Because of this we have designed and developed a colour-level lamp which enables people to tune a room to the required level of light and the best tone of that light. An infinite range of illumination is available to the person who has such an instrument to hand.

If one puts people into an area where there is too much light, a general introversion takes place. People will close up, become shy, will restrict their conversation and communication. When an area is lit too dimly people will become unsure, nervous, and again communication will be poor. They tend to make 'reassuring' noises, such as whistling or humming.

A gentle level of illumination with a centre from where the light issues is found to be of the greatest help – people can choose in such a room exactly where they wish to sit.

Under red illumination, vitality and physical excitement is enhanced – a red light in a room can be very good for lovemaking. On the other hand, a blue light distances objects, the mind expands and consciousness disappears; thus sleep invariably ensues. Sleep is, in fact, often made possible by the introduction of a blue light.

Yellow light has a tendency to cause detachment and an unpleasant feeling of not belonging. In cases where people are subjected to yellow light and a yellow environment, they may become utterly irresponsible. In January 1970 at an exhibition in London the following occurence was reported:

> ... exhibits in three rooms, one black, one green, one yellow. No trouble in the first two: in the yellow room all the objects are getting smashed up. What's not broken is pinched. Things were so bad last weekend the organisers thought they would have to close the show. Same vigilant attendants in all rooms; no obvious reason why vandalism should be confined to one room. Only explanation so far – colour: yellow incites the educated middle classes to violence!

From a report of experiments carried out by Hans Jenny, we can read the following: 'A downward stream of gas subjected to a constant vibration. The following veil of gas assumes a laminar pattern under the influence of sound. Eddy and wave formations also appear as turbulences.'

The finer and the more flexible a substance is, the more quickly it responds to sound or even light waves. The human body is such a finely tuned instrument that it responds instantaneously to all influences. The mental, emotional and finally physical responses to such influences can be either beneficial or detrimental; so the above gas is quickly 'manipulated' by sound into a predictable pattern. I am sure that as we proceed with our research we will be able to prove the extreme sensitivity of the human being to colour and sound as healing or sick-making influences. This suggests to us that here we have a highly sensitive body which responds to the sound almost instantaneously. A more solid body would take longer and would first have to move towards a state of flexibility before it could actually respond to the sound. From this we would deduce that a tungsten filament in an electric bulb moves with the vibration of electricity, $50+50$ (cycle under 240v), or $60+60$ (cycle under 100v). However, before it can become really mobile and respond to these cycles it heats up and glows; thus we have a steady light which we find corresponds to natural daylight to a high degree.

Many people are disturbed at the use of vapour-filled tube lights, strip lights or fluorescent lights. The sodium or mercury vapour responds directly to the vibrations of the electrical current and hence becomes an unsteady trembling light that has an unfavourable effect on the nervous system of humans, animals and plants. Even more serious effects are experienced when the lighting goes wrong, as it does frequently. It can flicker in the ratio of 7–12 cycles per second and in this particular area lies a brain rhythm known as the alpha waves. When a light flicker starts to approach the brain cycle of alpha, very uncomfortable feelings are generated. Finally, if these flickers become identical with those of an individual working under such a light, the person can be subjected to an artifically induced epileptic fit or seizure. This has never happened under tungsten illumination.

Many people complain of stomach ache or headaches when working under these lights, but the people's health is not often taken into account when economy is considered. All waves have effects upon all living matter; to some degree these waves raise or lower consciousness. People can be persuaded to get used to

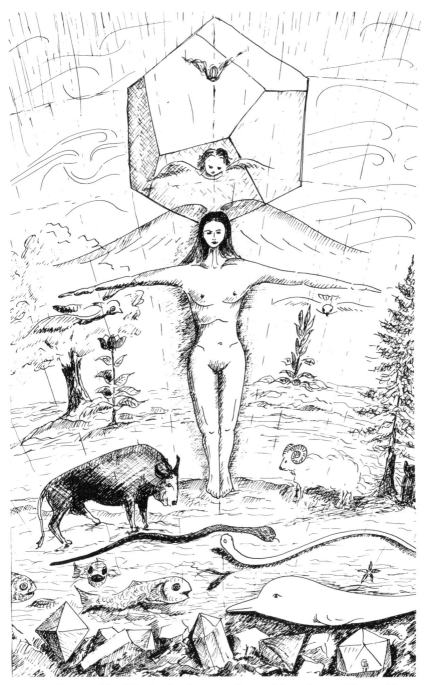

Man; Figure 4.8   The bridge between the visible and invisible world.

such influences and the effects of an environment designed only to satisfy economy for the sake of saving finance. But it is important to consider that economy is real only when we see the well-being of humans as the first consideration and part of economy in design and the total environment.

It can be said that the human being lives in his waking life predominantly on beta waves, the animal on alpha (unless raised to play or aggression). Plants have ceta waves predominantly, and minerals delta. (See Figure 4.9) It is man who, through meditation, can tap all these four states of consciousness (See Figure 4.8). There is as yet no drug which can evoke delta waves in people. It might be that such waves induced by drugs could kill the individual who partook of such a strong drug.

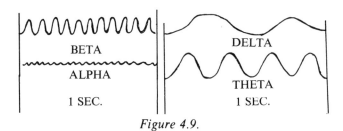

BETA

ALPHA

1 SEC.

DELTA

THETA

1 SEC.

Figure 4.9.

Chapter 5

The Human Spine as an Instrument of Sensitivity

Physicists know that in outer space appear trace elements which are so fine that they cannot materialise for any length of time, but that when slow enough vibrations are reduced gradually a very fine substance can change over to become visible and still be alive as a recording instrument. The human form is very much this kind of highly sensitive being, capable of so much more than originally believed. The spine is this wonder of creation.

I believe that all is eternal on the so-called invisible levels. In man's body is mirrored the ultimate vibration which through the inbuilt patterns and grids of energy can be a consciousness-enhanced being. For this to be possible the rhythms and proportions of the human skeleton are inevitably unique and it is not by chance that we are told 'So GOD created man in his own image . . .'.

Now in the downward flow of the vibrations we find this amazing picture: that man, although also visible, is, according to Teilhard de Chardin, the key to eternity of the whole cosmic creation by way of his memory. The study of proportions, the rhythms of metamorphosis of each bone, but particularly the spine, will reveal the secrets of responsive form, a recorder of what is in the invisible world inscribed as eternal creation. Long before this skeleton has actually become visible, unseen vibrations of colour, and previously light and originally darkness, have been responsible for creating, through low enough vibrations of sound, the traces of the mineral and fluid matter later found in the human spine and final form.

It is at that point that Rudolf Steiner suggests proceeding to a study of the finer rhythms in water and fire, scientifically. Hans Jenny took up the challenge at the time and carried out research into the effects of sound on all kinds of matter imaginable, from sand to iron filings and water to oils. It is in this area that the rhythms produce through the symphony of sound all the basic patterns which we can find in nature; and ultimately in the human spine and appending limbs.

All things are already in the original vibrations before these become manifest, through rhythms, in the visible world. The human spine contains some of the most beautiful and rhythmic progressions and metamorphoses that can be studied in visible matter; they are perhaps the most perfect reflections of the eternal law of form and, consequently, consciousness.

The human spine is a miracle of creation which has arisen out of sound. The metamorphosis which is seen in it can only be understood with a high degree of awe and wonder. While still in the womb this spine develops from the ovum, the sphere. Almost like a snail shell in spiral formation, it develops gradually to become the main structure on which the whole human posture is constructed.

The skull, retaining a very close resemblance to the original form of the ovum, is succeeded by the development of the various vertebrae. These change by degrees as we move down the spine from the atlas to the coccyx and sacrum. Each vertebra is a metamorphosis of its predecessor. When we look at this spine in the light of colour and sound, we can see that it is ordered into a series of five groups of eight bones.

The Five Groups of Vertebrae

Evolution of the spine is related to the five great kingdoms which we find spanning this visible world and the invisible area of what we may call here the divine world, which is not necessarily 'visible' to all at first. I suggest that there was once a time when man's body was not as dense as it is now and that during those early days much more was 'seen' by everyone.

Those who are concerned with human affairs today are usually led, in one way or another, to consider questions to which at first they have no answers. Some of us persist and find, individually, answers which can satisfy; others dismiss them as areas which do not belong to our work. I am now putting a view which is likely to answer some of the many questions and I would make it quite clear that these are not final answers, but serve only as a starting point for further investigation.

We can see that the first eight segments of the coccyx and sacrum correspond to the mineral kingdom and that the lumbar region, together with the last three dorsal vertebrae, can be seen to be the plant kingdom. The next section can be seen to correspond to the animal kingdom and the last section of the spine, first dorsal and all the cervicals, can be aligned with the human kingdom. The skull finally is, to me at least, the realm of the kingdom of the gods.

Posture

Our next consideration will be the whole of the human posture as seen from birth to adulthood. The child descends head downwards into the world at the moment of birth. The immediate changes which occur at this significant moment in the life of a human soul are adquately and most beautifully described in a book by a French gynaecologist, Frederick Leboyer.* From the time of birth the spine takes up an amount of stress which hitherto has been taken care of by the fluid inside the womb in which the body has been suspended. From this moment on it is dependent upon the care with which a mother handles the baby. Its predominant posture at this moment is horizontal and this posture should be noted as being of paramount importance to the mental and physical development of the growing being.

A sudden waking up is, even in adulthood, often a shock which causes the whole day to be out of rhythm. The gentle and gradual waking out of the sleep into day consciousness is the privilege that retains the sensitivity of a human being and, in my estimation, ensures good communication and orientation for the day. If that privilege is given at the start of a physically independent life (after birth) is should ensure the development of trust and love.

* *Birth Without Violence,* Wildwood House, 1975.

Our present civilisation will not overcome crime (aggression), violence and nervous breakdowns until we act according to the law of gentle, loving birth and let this experience be remembered every morning of our lives. This simple attitude to a day will ensure greater harmony to flow. The early months of a baby's existence are the morning of its life; and the deep sleep dawning into dream, the dream into visions, these into recognition and then into formulation and finally concepts must not be severed from each other so as to be unrelated floating bits of information – but retained as a coherent, unified concept of man and his environment. This need is most perfectly answered by not forcing a baby to sit up prematurely but by letting the movement develop naturally. Any speeding up of the process at this time will later on take its revenge in the life of that human being. The events which take place at this time of the development are closely connected with the later depth of consciousness of this person. To describe this adequately we should look at Figure 5.1. All the vibrations of the universe and those of the earth have an effect upon this body. The consciousness which later on enters the person is not present at this time.

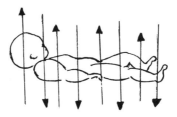

Figure 5.1.

Consciousness of being able to form and act upon concepts and understanding is another level of awareness which is, of course, essential to the individual who has reached maturity. Thus the gradual differentation of the various levels of consciousness accompanies the process of maturation in the human being. At the time of birth this consciousness is still far out in the space where the soul formed the intention to materialise. This universe, as it is called, is itself like a vast, as yet unmeasured, womb.

Out there in the far distances exist the relationships between the stars to which we are, in a mysterious way, all linked. Men may ignore this fact but deep down it calls up a feeling that we have an affinity with the constellations of all the signs of the zodiac.

The womb is an imitation of the universal laws governing all matter, from the geode or nodule in which are growing the crystals according to the energy patterns of the universe to the final complexity of the human womb where the most sensitive instrument, the human body, 'crystallises'. Because of its immeasurably fine sensitivity, it is also prone to upsets or breakdowns of its perfect working. We currently have an enormous amount of knowledge which shows this to be an irrefutable reality. During this early horizontal posture phase of the child's life, the memories of the vast world from which it has come gradually condense and the child is, in its mental process, forced to reverse the images which are until that moment still present as a faint reminder of the space without. It is not only the brain which is involved in this process of changing over but also the rest of the body. Indeed, all the glands are beginning to make new adjustments and it is these glands which later on contain much of the true human intelligence. Those who know something about clear and objective thinking, which is known in some circles as meditation, will know how vital the ductless glands are to the successful process of becoming a full human being through the use of these glands which are nothing more than further doors to fuller perception. Now we can begin to see how a sudden and thoughtless change from one experience into another is, in the newborn child, to be considered extremely dangerous. According to the gentleness and the protection, the patience and the love, we can devote to the child at that stage, it will later develop more fully as a person.

When we take into account how the consciousness in this position is really much closer to the animal world by virtue of the same spine position, we can see how from there we can only start to accomplish the human posture when the reversal process within the child is completed. From that moment on the child can stand upright and has great joy in doing just this. Now energies begin to concentrate and this is due to the vibrations which are no longer so widely cast over the length of the spine but drawn together into a much narrower band of space (see Figure 5.2)

Now that contact has been made with the forces of gravity, magnetism and energy are exchanged between the centre of universe (directly vertically above each being, whether human or not), and the centre of the earth, creating a very clear line of vibrations which are registered (received), translated and transmitted. Because of the sensitivity of the human instrument, the power of thought and reasoning arise out of this upright position.

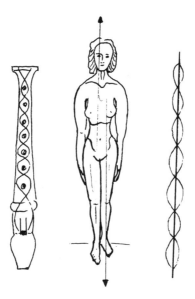

Figure 5.2.

The next step is that the child will begin to reverse the sounds which are heard. In other words, here we now have the phenomenon of the mirror, or the figure 8. When this is completed speech will become possible. It is only because of this concentration of the vibrations which now go through the human spine that the energies are called up which make available to the child the whole speech and sound world.

The last reversal is the reversal of colour. A child up to the age of about three years is still predominantly aware of the complementary colour; that is to say that if the child looks at a green lawn, the actual colour it sees is magenta and not green. For those who are interested in reading more deeply about the development of the child I would recommend the works of Dr Karl König and Rudolf Steiner. Because of the above phenomena the colours are also reversed and have to be relearned on the way to entering the visible world.

Gradually, because the upright posture is maintained for longer periods as the child grows up, consciousness arises ever more significantly; time makes use of space. In the course of the first twelve years of a human being's life on earth, there is an energy link between the earth's centre and the far-out regions of the universe. This is a complete communication of all the energies which we can experience, from the physical to the purely spiritual vibrations. It is in this uprightness of man that consciousness can arise as the concentration of the vibrations increases, being now filtered by a very narrow band or channel, instead of the more widely cast space, which is the case in man's sleeping position and the general posture of animals.

Now we can see how this comparatively narrow band of vibrating energy flows through the body of man. At each of the ductless glands it raises, in its up and down flow, another tone and another colour combination according to the chemistry which this particular body is producing. This chemistry is a very personal one and depends a great deal on the food intake, the environmental influences, the emotional state and even the thought patterns of the individual.

I mentioned just now that there is both a musical and a colour resonance as the interplay of vibrations, or better, radiations, are playing the instrument called the human body, or for that matter any physical body, even that of a stone. It is said that the tensions, together with the actual fibre of a string, produce the particular colouring of the sound which is obtained when the string is moved. Thus the interaction of the radiation is related to the human person; each time the string is played it has a general, permanent sound, a temporary sound and a momentary sound. In this way we can now begin to see that there will be no repeat pattern possible and that the highly responsive nervous system of a human being changes continually.

The Spine: Colour, Sound and the Signs of the Zodiac

Nevertheless, there is a general pattern underlying this living, developing and fluctuating response. Because of this we can put a measure to the colour and the sounds which we can detect in the human spine (see Figure 5.3 and Colour Plate 8 between pages 84 and 93). This column of light and sound is the link which is capable of channelling the earth vibrations and the cosmic energies and, by playing on them together, raise in man the level of consciousness and consequent activities.

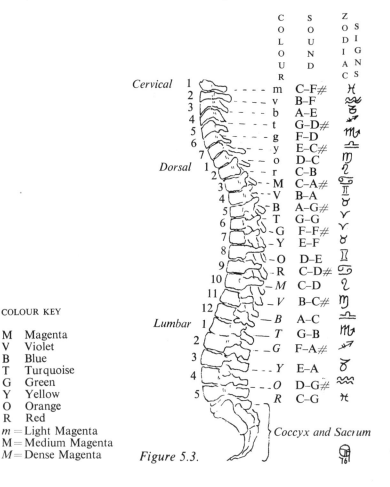

COLOUR KEY

M   Magenta
V   Violet
B   Blue
T   Turquoise
G   Green
Y   Yellow
O   Orange
R   Red
m = Light Magenta
M = Medium Magenta
M = Dense Magenta

Figure 5.3.

It is through the spine that we experience the reactions which come from the brain and branch out into the nerves which issue from the spine at intervals. From the womb, or geode, in this case the brain, down to the last part of the spine, the nerves serve an ever-increasingly more physical function and finally end up providing for the actual basic needs for the maintenance of 'the instrument'.

These intervals are carefully measured and move downwards in a harmonic progression. The sound of each vertebra follows a descending scale as these increase in volume. The colouring of this sound depends on the actual form of each vertebra.

The divisions we find are in three parts; cervical, dorsal and lumbar. The complete numbers of each section are also a very beautiful harmonic progression (see Figure 5.4). To make a

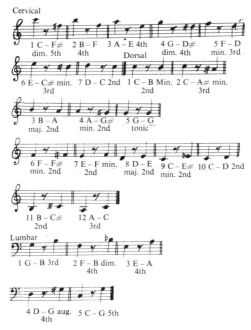

Figure 5.4.

NOTE: This scale of intervals is derived from the ascending diatonic C major scale and the descending chromatic scale. Both scales synchronise on the G above middle C (at 256 c. per sec.).

vibration more significant and lend more strength to it, we find that we have the following order rather than a logical one: 7 – 12 – 5. The 7 and the 5 make up the second 12, being the twelve dorsal vertebrae.

We can also compare this number arrangement with the known fact that man has five outer senses and seven main ductless glands. To each of these ductless glands can be attributed another meaning. In the work of Rudolf Steiner we find that he suggests there are twelve senses in the human being – the well-known five and the less well-known inner senses which are seven in number. Thus twelve is a very interesting number, which we could discuss for many chapters; and even in this chapter we shall encounter it frequently.

The vibrations found in the field of sound production (music) are not significant for the human spine merely by chance. Both the string and the wind instruments are represented in principle. Clearly, a spine looks very much like a recorder (see Figure 5.5); the sound is the spinal fluid which rises and falls with the activities of the brain, the breath of the lungs and the calmness, or otherwise, of the heart. We can certainly say that there is, albeit inaudible, music played all through the life of a human being that seems to use this instrument, the spine, as its body of resonance.

The recorder, an instrument that registers

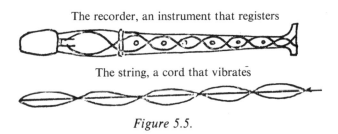

The string, a cord that vibrates

Figure 5.5.

All dance forms are derived from the sacred temple dances. They have, as has so much else, lost more and more of their original meaning, the art of understanding why and how a rhythm is significant to each dance and its application to the body. All dances originally maintained contact with the universal rhythms. They ensured that the life-energy was as near possible conducted into the body. However, the body is too dense in its fluid and mineral content for this to be entirely successful, so the dances were directed towards healing as part of the temple activities. Today's dance forms are almost detrimental to health. We can see now a complete reversal of the original meaning of dance.

It is time for us to reinterpret the meaning of dance and movement. This is what we can see today in the attempts of Eurythmy, a form of dance re-conceived by Rudolf Steiner and Professor Bernhard, Wosin and many others. Eventually it will again fulfil its original task and, because of its period of debasement, a heightened level of consciousness.

The Spine and the Law of Gravity

It is important to consider how the proportions of the spine are related to the law of gravity. Stand in a level field, throw a stone and then measure its flight. (This can be done by filming the flight of the stone.) We will find that the stone has apparently a very even curve of ascent and descent. The evenness is there, but the actual picture we get is that of a wave. This wave displays a very significant form. It rises on a straight incline and then levels off before finally falling steeply to the ground. The law of gravity of the stone being thrown can now be translated into the proportions of the three areas of the spine as in Figure 5.6. The figures given are in the proportions of the golden mean. If we now measure the three changes of direction the stone makes we arrive at the measurements of $8 - 5 - 3$, rise, levelling off and fall.

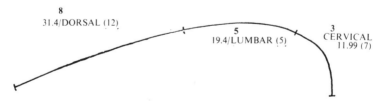

Figure 5.6   The flight path of a stone in relation to the proportionate lengths of the three sections of the spine.

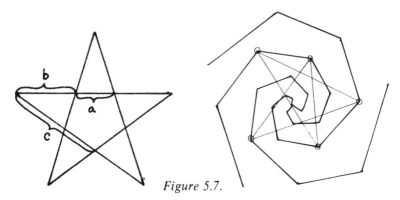

Figure 5.7.

The tracing of the midpoint of each rib of a cabbage reveals that there is an albeit irregular pentagram seen in the inter-relationship between points. Taking the human hand and half closing it, we find the same proportions, and the same irregularity. The perfect is only in the unseen and not in the materialised field. (*See also Plate 2* opp. page 84.)

The spine and all natural things like plants and shells obey the rhythms and proportions of the golden mean and it is like a well written drama. (Details of this can be found in H.E. Huntley: *The Divine Proportion, a Study in Mathematical Beauty* Dover Publications Inc., New York, 1970.

When we find that three very diverse teachings come together to support the same idea, we are compelled to give the subject further thought. Regarding the human spine we find that mathematics, music and Chinese ancient philosophy all point to the same conclusions. The teaching of the Tao, ancient in its origin and therefore very close to the beginning of man's wisdom, has become blurred by time and the loss of that wisdom; but we can retrieve a general picture.

We have to resort to the foundation principle of man, as with the Qabalah. A he is not a he nor is a she a she, unless we have the complementary energies working together. The reader should cast aside the old ingrained sex differentiation and look at the distribution of the energies as being of the earth (intuitive, mother nature) on one hand, and the intellect (logical, father nature) on the other. We have in the spine two scales: our analysis tells us that there are three diatonic scales playing against the two chromatic scales. Following this up with the natural semitones we find that, at the three gates which the Chinese in their Tao teaching offer as gates of renewal or offering, in the musical progression of the intervals we come to what I can only call a 'little dance', which is performed before each gate as a gesture to allow entry, a thanksgiving to the gatekeeper. Possibly this may seem to be merely a beautiful image – but the implications of the image are too important to be disregarded.

When we look at the co-ordination chart (Table 5.1) giving all the musical and the coloured scales, we must study them one by one, and yet remember that only by considering them as a whole can we begin to make a sensible, meaningful picture.

Table 5.1 draws together the major correlations so far discussed in connection with the human spine, sound, colour, the C major scale and the chromatic scale. Taking the semitones in groups of twelve, we arrive at the exact points which in the Tao are marked as 'Gates'. There are three places where this happens and one could say that these are a kind of loop. In column 2 are added the eight bones making up the skull and the eight bones making up the sacrum. The coccyx is the ninth bone. It is my firm belief that this bone is again subdivided into 8 + 1 and that this continues *ad infinitum*. Maybe this is symbolic of the eternal being of man.

We begin with the densest of the colours, red. This colour has a vibratory rate of $4 \cdot 6 \times 10^{14}$. In layman's terms this is $4 \cdot 6$ trillions per second. Orange and yellow follow and go into the white light. On this rising scale we have to do with the male energy in colour. Green cannot manifest without the female scale of violet. Blue (the least dense colour, vibrating at $7 \cdot 5 \times 10^{14}$) and turquoise scales descend and end again in the white light(*). Only through the interaction of these two scales can the green arise. Green appears three times in the spine when you look at the table. In each of those places is found a very fine point of balance which has a certain effect on the human posture.

In our investigation using the above-mentioned colours we discovered that green represents physical balance and stability, and turquoise tranquillity and calmness. Thus there must be a

Chapter Five

TABLE 5.1
CO-ORDINATION CHART

Predominantly Descending, Feminine ♀ —

	0	1	2	3	4	5	
WATER	12/12	C	(8)	C	ULTRA	C maj.	1,024 c per sec.
AIR	13/12	B	1	C	M	dim. 9th	
INTUITIVE SCALE	13/12	A⁺	2	B	V	dim. 9th	
	12/12	A	3	A	B	A maj.	
	11/12	G⁺	4	G	T	dim. 8th	
	10/12	G	5	F	G	dom. 7th	
I. *scale of 8 colours*	10/12	F⁺	6	E	Y	dim. 7th	
	9/12	F	7	D	O	A⁺ maj.	
	8/12	E	1	C	R	C maj.	
Generally blue	9/12	D⁺	2	C	M	G⁺ maj.	512 c per sec.
spectrum	9/12	D	3	B	V	G maj.	
	8/12	C⁺	4	A	B	A maj.	
	7/12	C	5	G	T	C maj.	
II. *Balanced*	6/12	B	6	F	G	dim. 5th	
scale of 8 colours	6/12	A⁺	7	E	Y	dim. 5th	
	5/12	A	8	D	O	D maj.	
	4/12	G⁺	9	C	R	G⁺ maj.	
Intervals downwards,	5/12	G	10	C	M	C min.	
unwinding	5/12	F⁺	11	B	V	B min.	
	4/12	F	12	A	B	F min.	
	3/12	E	1	G	T	C min.	
Left side of spine,	3/12	D⁺	2	F	G	D⁺ min.	
chromatic scale	2/12	D	3	E	Y	A min.	
III. *Dense*	1/12	C⁺	4	D	O	D min.	
scale of 8 *colours*	0	C	5	C	R	tonic	128 c per sec
	1/12	(B)	(8)	(C)	INFRA	C min.	

Predominantly Ascending, Masculine 0

FIRE
EARTH
LOGICAL SCALE (diatonic), right side of spine
Generally red spectrum · intervals upwards, stimulating (tension)

Figure 5.8.

KEY
* = White light
0 = Steps in semitones between intervals
1 = The chromatic scale
2 = The number of vertebrae:
    1–7 cervical
    1–12 dorsal
    1–5 lumbar
3 = The diatonic scale
4 = The colours: R – red, O – orange, Y – yellow, G – green, T – tourquoise, B – blue, V – violet, M – magenta
5 = Major keys, minor keys; dim – diminished, dom – dominant.

very fine balance for the human upright posture. This has been discussed with osteopaths and chiro-practitioners, who in the course of their studies have found the above assumption to be absolutely accurate, and are very pleased to find correlation and verification of their findings.

Taking now the other side of the colour scales and reducing the darkness between the red and the violet, we arrive at the other 'created' colour which is magenta. When a man and woman find a level of communication on the soul level and not on the physical level, between them they reduce density. In other words darkness and this spiritual colour appear. (It can actually be found through meditation.) Each spectrum, all five of them, is complete in itself and must always culminate in magenta. In a way we can say there has been a physical meeting in the green and a spiritual meeting in the magenta. Both of these are valid experiences which have their echo in the spine of man.

A friend, who travels a lot in the South Sea islands, told me that the natives there use the human spine as an instrument to evoke compelling sounds for ritual dances. From this account I have become very interested in the connection between the spine and the sound of the whole human skeleton.

What Sounds Does a Spine Make?

Among studies done so far on sound and form I have been interested in the work of Chladni and Jenny. From this it seems evident that the forms in our environment are frozen sound. The communications I have had with Anne Macauley and Maria Renold-Neusheller have also been the bases for this research. In as much as we can link sound to the human form, it must be remembered that the modern concert pitch is not necessarily the true pitch which the universal energies use to compose the forms, which we can see after these have manifested themselves through the sound–matter interaction.

From A. Macauley's work I deduce that the sounds G and F sharp can easily be linked to some of the bones in even a living body: G for the skull and F sharp for the cheekbone. It may be that the actual sound is not right if we compare present

COMPARISON BETWEEN WEIGHT AND PITCH OF
VERTEBRAE IN FEMALE AND MALE SPINES

	Female			*Male*		
1	2	3	1	2	3	
1c	0·3125	C 1,024				Basic pitch used
2c	0·3750	D				= 256 c per sec.
3c	0·1250	A				c = cervical
4c	0·1250+	C 1,024				d = dorsal
5c	0·1250	G				l = lumbar
6c	0·1875−	F♯				
7c	0·3125	C 1,024				
1d	0·2500+	A	1d	0·5000	A♭	
2d	0·2500	G♯	2d	0·4375	G	
3d	0·1875+	A♯	3d	0·4375	G	From here down-
4d	0·1875	G	4d	0·4375+	A♭	wards the sounds
5d	0·1875	F	5d	0·5000	G♯	are very much
6d	0·2500−	D	6d	0·5000	G♯	clearer
7d	0·2500	E	7d	0·5625	A♯	
8d	0·2500+	F	8d	0·5625	G♯	
9d	0·3125	G	9d	0·6250	G	
10d	0·3125	C 256	10d	0·6875	C 512	
11d	0·3125	B	11d	0·7500−	G♯	
12d	0·3125+	A	12d	0·7500+	G	
1l	0·4375+	G	1l	0·9375	G♯	
2l	0·5000	G	2l	1·1250	G	
3l	0·5625	F♯	3l	1·2500	F	
4l	0·5625	F	4l	1·2500	G♯	
5l	0·6250	G	5l	missing – possibly diseased		

NOTE:
As there were only $\frac{1}{16}$ oz weights available:
  − = slightly less than recorded weight   *Figure 5.9.*
  + = slightly more

concert pitch with the original pitch universally used by J. S. Bach and his contemporaries, and even by some more recent composers. From research currently in progress on 'perfect pitch' in relation to perfect colour memory, we have found that many who have written in (310 people have contacted us so far and it is still early days) claiming perfect pitch actually say that they have to transpose music when they hear it on radio or records. Evidently they must be linking back to the C = 256 c. per sec. This is the original pitch, still used today by the medical profession for hearing tests, etc. These claims have led me finally to acquire an unarticulated spine and check each vertebra for sound and weight, using the pitch middle C = 256 c. per sec. Concert pitch is 8 c. per sec. higher than what is known as Pythagorean pitch.

Table 5.2 shows the results of an experiment conducted on a female spine, cleaned and prepared for study at the School of Medicine, Bristol University, Department of Anatomy, on 4 March 1976.

An identical check was made on an incomplete male spine – none of the cervical vertebrae was available – found in the open and not prepared for medical research.

When the doctor in charge of this research brought to me the remains of this young man's skeleton, he said that the police had brought it in from somewhere near Bristol and he personally thought it was the spine of a twenty-year-old man. The weights of the vertebrae as given in column 2 may be meaningful not only in relation to the sound but also to the study of balance of the spine as a column of support for human posture.

This chart can now be linked and compared with the charts on pages 92, 116 and 119. There are, of course, discrepancies as we will not find all the answers at once. It is in such incompatibilities that our research often has its origin.

Dating by Dowsing

Dowsing is an art which has been used in recent times by advanced scientific departments to obtain information about objects or in areas where there is at present no other clue to go by. It cannot be used as evidence in a court but can lead to evidence. This art, if you like to call it an art, has gradually been growing in my own field of research. I am never surprised if I am already, through dowsing, in possession of information I later discover by very laborious and time-consuming work with the conventional methods of research. My own way of dowsing is using my left middle finger over a map or chart and I receive small, (electrical) impulses which tell me that there is a flaw or a point to ask questions. When I have received an impulse I then start asking questions such as: 'Is it the liver?' When the answer is 'yes' I get another impulse, if 'no' there is no impulse. This can be used to find out when, where and sometimes how, by a process of elimination. Not using a pendulum for me works better and quicker.

The following is a description of a particular experience I had and illustrates my personal approach to research into fields that entail the use of bones, living plants or any living matter. This approach, to me at least, lends the investigator a kind of protection from unwanted, unbalanced influences.

In any research I undertake, I say 'thank you' to any matter with which I happen to be working at the time. In the case of a human being I quietly acknowledge the divinity of that being. Even the remains of a once-living person are treated with the same respect.

On 5 March 1976 at 2.30 a.m. I awoke and found myself 'receiving' the following message:

> I, who once used this spine, was twenty-two years of age. I died fifteen years ago. I was a shop assistant at Gardiner's of Bristol (a large ironmongers in that city). I did not die a natural death.

After this the message, such as it was, faded out.

Chapter 6

Practical Advice on using Colour to treat Illness

Attitude to the Patient

This chapter is intended to offer some practical advice to the colour therapist. Much thought must go into the preparation of all the instruments, the environment in which we work, the furnishings and the actual materials we use to create the congenial surroundings in which we can receive a patient and work harmoniously with him or her. Obviously the colours and the textures are important.

How should you conduct your own self? You will say to the patient that you have absorbed considerable knowledge in order to be useful, conscientious and discreet. Remember that ulti-mately the patient will expect to know everything that is happening to him or her. Do not rush anything but adopt the attitude of listening most carefully. You will be 'told' when to say the things which the patient can cope with, and what these are. In moments of doubt, say nothing and consult the team of doctors you are working with.

It is better for the patient to know what is wrong with him/her; the effect it will have is usually a matter of timing and the love with which you communicate. A patient who knows what is wrong and is assured of your and the doctor's constant support can fight his or her condition very well, and in every case much better than if he or she were left in uncertainty. Uncertainty arises in all cases where the patient is left to guess, where pretty words and benevolent attitudes try and hide the true picture from him/her.

One cannot stress enough the importance of your thoughts

whilst you work for your patient. The things which you cannot say on a certain day and you feel ought to be said must actually be said as soon as possible after the patient has left the room. In this moment you must concentrate and address yourself to the higher being of this person, and in the clearest terms available to you speak to the soul as if its owner were present. You will be surprised how often, at the next meeting, the ground is already prepared so well that you can say what is important then. Invariably, in my own experience, it is actually the patient who will begin to speak about the question or the subject which was so difficult to broach before.

Those who work with a pendulum to get their diagnosis and the treatment right ought to make sure that they truly comprehend this method, that there is no fumbling about whether or not to use such an aid. It boils down to getting information from the most reliable source. I would advise the student to obtain helpful booklists and advice from the relevant society.*

The Basic Requirements for a Therapy Room (for colour, massage and scanning)

Starting with the floor, it is important that this is made of wood or stone, although cement will do. Avoid plastic tiles and covers such as nylon carpets. Wool is acceptable and up to 20 per cent nylon can be used. The carpet should be blue or turquoise and the felt or undercarpet not of rubber but of a conducting material such as cork, paper, or paper or cloth felt.

The walls should be painted in a cobalt blue non-gloss, possibly even a non-emulsion paint (though this is difficult to get these days). The ceiling needs to be of a lighter colour and should preferably bear the design shown in Figure 6.1. The ceiling lights must be non-glare and on a dimmer switch; otherwise wall lights are best.

The general effect of such a room will be to relax the patient, giving hope for future life by the figure-of-eight with its pro-

* The Secretary, The British Dowsers' Association, 19 High Street, Eydon, Daventry NN11 6PP, England.

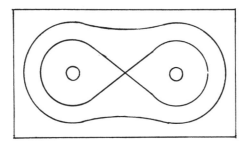

Figure 6.1   Design for a ceiling.

tective form and the clarity of being centred in the midpoints of each lobe of the figure 8. To help any room to have a peaceful atmosphere, the corners of the wall and ceiling relationship may need to have their normal angles changed to help meet the need for protection.

A basin and water should be available; also a cubicle in which to undress, and a white garment for the patient to wear in order to allow any colour to be used without interference from other shades. If possible the actual source of light should be natural; thus we can use existing windows and make a frame for the various filters, enabling us to shut off and alternate the colours.

It has been found that nylon cord and good polished tubing (glass tubing bent to the correct angles may be used) can provide very smooth and silent shutter operation. There should be sixteen different filters for the actual colour therapy.

When the colour-ray lamps, or local illuminator, are used then it will be necessary to leave the rest of the room in a gentle blue light. Blue, of all the colours, accommodates the rest of the spectrum most willingly.

A colour-level lamp for evening, morning or night treatment, or even, in the winter time, during the day, will be useful. When daylight is not available, electric lights may be used. These should be fitted behind the filter over the window.

The actual 'box' can be made to measure, to fit into the window frame, if necessary. In a room where the window is not suitable for this, electric light will have to be used, although daylight is infinitely better (and cheaper).

COLOUR-RAY LAMPS

This instrument is specially designed to offer to the patient a local colour exposure which is otherwise not possible. It can be set so that the beams of light are focused on or inside the body when the treatment is needed (see Figure 6.2).

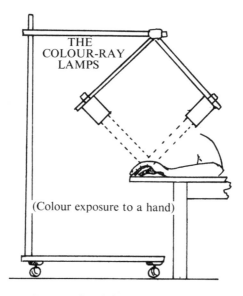

THE COLOUR-RAY LAMPS

(Colour exposure to a hand)

Figure 6.2   Colour-ray lamps.

The left filter will, in each case, remain unchanged as regards the selected colours (see colour filter numbers on page 000). The right filter will have, in addition, the two extra numbers: 17 for the blue range and 9 for the red. This ensures stimulation and therefore a much better reaction to the treatment. There may be the need to treat a number of times in accordance with the advice of the doctor in charge, or a single treatment may suffice if the case is cleared, as can happen, after the treatment of 24¼ minutes.

This instrument is very carefully set up so as to use only a minimum of electric light. It has been found that if we use very strong lights, the electromagnetic field set up around the instrument more often than not interferes with the benefit of the coloured light.

APERTURES

The apertures for the colour therapy windows are important. The light which enters through these openings carries not only the colour but also the form. The effect which an aperture has is to reverse the outer image, as is well known by people who are concerned with optics (see Figure 6.3).

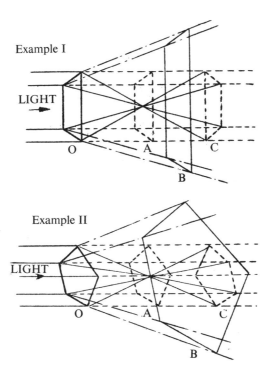

KEY

O = The actual window through which the light is admitted
A = Sunlight, which would travel parallel
B = The speed of light through the original window
C = The reversal of the outer image and the grid of different light intensities where light actually creates the pools of differentiated degrees of brightness

Figure 6.3   The three effects of light shining through a window (aperture).

According to the shape of the aperture (see Figure 6.4), the light which shines into the therapy room has a certain structure by virtue of the 'grid' each different shape produces. Considering very fine influences is important. Again, it has to do with what we have termed the male and the female forms. Thus there are pools of concentrated light and pools of less intensive light within each form. These are very closely linked to the two complementary forms mentioned earlier, working here in co-operation. See Figure 6.5 for an example of a light 'grid'.

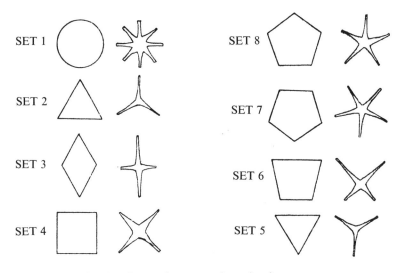

Set 5 to 8 uses the same colours but in reverse order. The two supplementary filters are 17 for the blue range and 9 for the red range of treatment and complementary colours.

SET	COLOUR NUMBER	COLOUR NAMES
1	6/16	primary red blue-green
2	35/19	deep golden amber dark blue
3	1/25	yellow/purple
4	39/13	primary green magenta

Figure 6.4   Apertures of the Colour Therapy **Windows.**

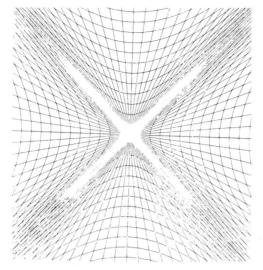

This particular design is appropriate to high energy physics, because it involves various features of the light cone and the time and space light directions, the light cone itself, of course, being associated with the darker and heavier lines.

Figure 6.5   Example of a light 'grid'.

CONSTRUCTION OF 'MALE WINDOWS'
There is no acute end to these points of these shapes. In fact at the 15×15 inch size the points works out at about ½ inch width.

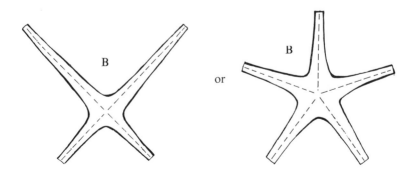

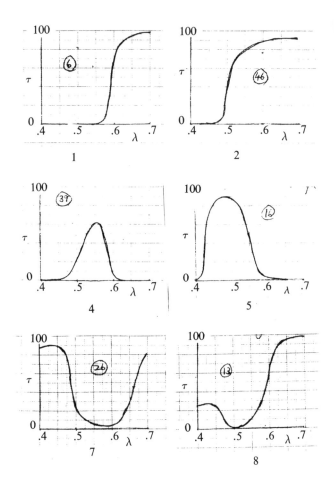

Diagnosis Using the Spine Chart

To develop colour treatment for therapeutic purposes, it is necessary to use the human spine for diagnostic purposes and learn to make sensitive the middle finger (preferably) of your left, sometimes right, hand. Take the colour-sound spine chart (Colour Plate 3, page 92) and lay it before you: now slowly move your middle finger from the base of the skull to the sacrum and coccyx, holding it about ½–¾ inches from the chart. You

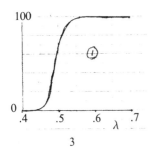

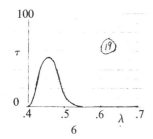

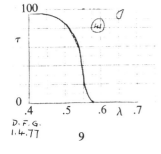

The eight wavelengths for the colours used in the colour-ray beamer plus working light and tinted filters.

No. 1   primary red
No. 2   orange (chrome yellow)
No. 3   yellow
No. 4   green
No. 5   turquoise (blue-green)
No. 6   dark blue
No. 7   purple (violet)
No. 8   magenta
No. 9   bright blue (working light)
No. 10   pale lavender (alteration filter)
No. 11   light rose (alteration filter)

λ = wavelength in UM
τ = % transmission

Figure 6.6   Wavelengths of the Eight Colour Filters.

will need to hold in your mind the name of the person whose illness you hope to diagnose, the age and sex. In the case of diagnosis of illness in an absent person you need to know, in addition to this, exactly where he/she is. Be sure that you know the full name. If there is a nickname by which this person is know, you need to know this too. Have at hand a pencil/paper to record at once the places which you think are affected. There will be at least two, usually three or more vertebrae which are out of true. Certainly one will be dominant, and this will be

129

cause of the present disease, underline the most prominent of the affected vertebrae.

How you register identification of the vertebrae varies from person to person. Often there is a kind of tickling feeling, as if an electric current is sparking from a certain vertebra to your finger. Make sure you do not touch the chart; if you do you will shortcircuit the vibrations, in which case you must start again from the top after earthing your finger. This you do by touching natural stone, metal, wood or earth, or woollen carpet over wood. Make sure you are not working on nylon or manmade fibre carpets, or plastic tiles. If this is unavoidable, you need to 'transmute' this artificial floor covering very consciously before you start. If you do not do this you will get wrong 'readings' through your finger, or none at all.

Go over the spine colour-sound chart at least three times. Keep your mind clear and receptive, trying not to prejudge in any way. Do not let the patient tell you first if she/he happens to know what is wrong or thinks she/he does. After consultation and checking completely, earth yourself and return the energies you have been tapping to state of equilibrium.

Compose yourself into the state of peace, linked with your higher self, and make contact with your God. Ask that the will of this God be done and not your own will. Enclose yourself with the one for whom you wish to be the channel for healing in an orb of thought and aura-ether, so that you can share all the vibrations.

The Three-Dimensional Orb

Look at Figure 6.5. Area A denotes the etheric sheath which in normal circumstances measures about 3–4½ inches all round the physical body of a human being. The next sheath is B and has the size of an orb which is approximately as large as a human being can stretch all round his body. This is the size of the aura which can be seen by some trained people. There is another field which is, however, much finer and is practically invisible.

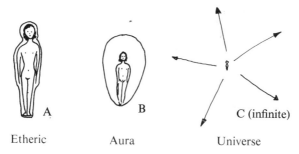

Etheric   Aura   Universe

Figure 6.7   The three sheaths surrounding the human body.

The next and final area C is as large as the thought field of the person, reaching out into the farthest places of this planet and indeed to the stars and the galaxies. This orb you fill with the being of God and yourself from your heart centre during therapy.

Make an image of the most perfect health, love and completeness that you are capable of. God is not young nor old, neither a man nor a woman. That being is perfection, absolute and eternal, and can only exist in the subtle life-field of the etheric world. Christ, Buddha and those who are said to be 'the ascended masters' have all returned to the state of God and are 'perfect' with all the attributes that are attached to this state of being. (See Theo Gimbel, *The Power of the Third*, Hygeia Publications, 1975.) God, Christ, the Spirit, the Eternal Being, all are ultimately that which we wish to become and with which we make an effort to identify.

In the early stages of work, and as often as you can, have a basin at hand with water and a towel, and perform the following rite:

(a)   touch the basin for earthing;
(b)   rinse your hands to return all impure density to the water;
(c)   dry your hands, letting the air absorb all density of a gaseous nature;
(d)   feel your warmth returning to your hands and let the fire burn up all unwanted matter;

(e) very fine energies lie above the four elements and we can balance out all remaining densities by offering those to the Ether.

After this you should be fully restored to your own nature; in fact you will often feel very refreshed.

It is most important to control your thoughts, since thoughts work instantaneously. Things happen as you order your consciousness which are vital. First of all, *never* make a judgement about any person with whom you wish to work. In the healing work he/she is equal to you and never anything else. Rather, let yourself be a mirror and ask silently what are the reflections he/she is making in your mirror. Ask very clear questions. These will arise out of the findings you have made on the colour-sound spine chart. You must, of course, have a good knowledge of anatomy and know which part of the spine is connected with which organs via the nervous system. Always ask via the heart first, and confirm via the brain secondly. The following procedure is now necessary.

1 You have connected yourself with the patient in the triple orb described above.
2 You are now a mirror.
3 Let that mirror be clear by putting none of your own ideas in the way.
4 Read without prejudice (this becomes more difficult as you get to know your patient; hence you have to guard against this). It becomes easier when you reinvite God into the orb.
5 Keep careful notes on each finding, with date, hour of day and weather condition, e.g. cold, raining, dry, warm, hot, etc.
6 Discuss your findings with the patient in a manner which demonstrates in every respect self-control and capacity to handle *all* you communicate.
7 Give a task to the patient which will provoke the right kind of thoughts and feelings. 'Have a plant in your house, look after it every morning and evening, see its life depending on yours, it is a captive in your hands, just as you are a captive in the love, light and life of God. Take care to love it, water it, but not too much nor too little. Give to this plant your breath, which contains for the

plant necessary foods, though to you they are a poison.'
Or: 'Paint or draw every day a picture with certain colours
and forms which are more helpful than others (wax
crayons are useful). However, make sure that a certain
amount of the complementary colour is also part of the
task. The picture need not be finished in one or two days
– set about it slowly.'

The consultant should find out the sort of things the
patient can do when the task is in hand and a few
consultations later you can ask: 'What are the thoughts
that this task provokes?' Talk about holding life in one's
own hands, the patient often thinks only you are capable
of doing anything. Return to him/her the confidence that
positive action provokes, which will lead to positive feeling
and, in the end, positive thoughts again.

8   With a qualified doctor, after discussion and verification
of your findings (you must accept the medical trained
person's comments and teaching), you both may feel that
a colour therapy course of, say, between three and nine
treatments is recommended. Your records should be made
available to all the medical team who are working together
on behalf of this particular patient.

In my thoughts, at this moment, a figure 8 will be appearing,
my physical finger being at the cross-point of this psychic figure
of 8. I myself ask for Christ's power of healing, that what is
present as wrong density in this body I am checking may be
both illuminated and made 'transparent', and that what is not
ready to be transmuted or healed is earthed for future trans-
mutation into light. I also make sure that I say 'Thy will be
done', not my own, often misguided, will. I am always aware
that some density or illness within each human being is there
to help in the work of the creator and we must transmute it in
our own way, remembering the illness is there for a good reason.
Therefore we must not remove the complaint without thought
for its purpose. But, at some moments, one 'receives the message'
that it is now the right time – that one may be the channel
through which can pour the healing power of Christ. May I add
that this also works for Buddhists, Moslems, Jews or any others
with sincere faith in their God, who have each their own image

of the supreme light. I have never liked the *flinging* off of density or illness and, by watching many healers, I have wrestled with this concept until I discovered the above-described figure 8 as a renewal symbol, or a balancing-out gesture. It comes from the work of Pythagoras, the School of Plato, where these energy patterns were known by way of the study of the sacred geometry.

I used to work with a pendulum, to which Bruce Macmanaway introduced me as far back as 1967. To him I owe so much, and many times he has helped me further just by saying the right thing at the right moment. Through him I also met Elizabeth Baerlein and Lavender Dower.* With them, in numerous discussions, I constantly learn more. I have since discarded my pendulum, but have found instead that my finger tips are able to register just as easily. It is particularly the middle finger of the left hand which responds most in my own field. Not being a very good medical student, I cannot identify the vertebrae of the spine in the flesh, so I resort to the colour-sound spine chart.

Colour Therapy: a Case Study

Colour therapy is more complete with the co-operation of a music therapist – hence you could discuss with this person the intervals which you have found via the colour-sound spine chart. A therapeutic melody can be composed to accompany the colour therapy sessions. You may be able to do this yourself, but it is not ideal. You must, as a colour therapist, understand the basic elements of music, but you may not be able to handle both the colour and the sounds at the same time. You can learn the tune by heart and sing it during the colour treatment. That is one way. However, a good music therapist can use a guitar and voice, whilst you work on the colour rhythms.

Here are some examples of colour therapy and music therapy working together:

---

* The Keys Trust.

CASE (1)

Asthma: Blue-violet-blue, alternating with deep orange-red-orange.

Spine:	C6 – yellow	E–C
	D2+D9 – magenta/	C–A (C=512)
	red	C–D (C=256)
	L3 – yellow	E–A

This turns out not to be an asthma case, but first treat as if for asthma. Many health problems are in fact psychosomatic conditions which, when the mental and emotional blocks are overcome, will allow the return of health of the patient. In this case we note that there is no blue nor any of the blue spectrum colours. These are needed and the therapist will have to work out the complementary colours to work on the patient. Thus the case looks as follows:

+ Yellow III	Violet I
+Red III	Turquoise I
−Magenta II	Green II
−Yellow I	Violet III

Choose your apertures for the colours. There are two colours which you will take if, as in this case, asthma is the 'complaint'. Asthma is in fact no longer the main cause for concern; there is a much more likely case for arthritis. So there will be a double treatment going on. First of all remove the asthmatic condition, which should be easy. The patient will be in the colour therapy room quickly falling asleep, several times, say three or four, a week. If at the end of, say, 20 minutes, the sleep has been free each time from any asthmatic attack, the therapist can verbalise as follows: 'You already know that the attacks were at night. Now I have proved that you can go to sleep and suffer no attack.' The asthmatic condition was due to a mental image which caused a psychosomatic asthma. Most patients (in my experience all) will soon realise that they have fallen asleep and woken up through the colour rhythms. It is the colour rhythms which induce the sleep. *Never* tell them you want them to go to sleep; this can only be discussed in retrospect.

However, you now know that the patient suffers, maybe lightly, from an arthritic condition. Refer back to your chart and prepare another treatment.

++ dominant impulse
−− minor impulse

A practical approach A patient, female, aged thirty-four, complains of asthma. She is sent for colour therapy by the doctor to the colour therapist. The general treatment colour for asthma is cobalt blue. This must, however, be adapted to suit the patient; it may need to have a little more red or a little more green in it.

We use the aperture of blue. This colour will then be used to alternate with orange, using the appropriate aperture (See chapter 5).

A No.42 and a No.43 will be overlaid for the blue, and a No. 5 for orange.

TREATMENT RHYTHMS

The shutters will be operated according to the timetable given below.

The blue shutter is open as soon as the patient enters the therapy room and during the preliminaries, including a possible change of clothes. A white dressing-gown should be made available to the patient and he/she should not wear any coloured underwear as this will influence the colours used. The garment should be of cotton, silk (not artificial) or wool material – not any of the manufactured fibres.

Have time for the patient. Do not hurry anything. Be precise with the colour therapy treatment itself.

During this treatment we suggest that healing music is played, ideally a guitar – live music. Otherwise a good 'untreated' tape specially recorded for such therapy is advisable.

Be prepared to offer advice after the treatment, which may be called counselling. A human soul may be made responsive and so the need to talk arises. As a colour therapist you should accept this challenge and use it during the time the treatment lasts. The timing used is not so much a measure as a rhythm that gradually relaxes the mental, emotional and physical state of the person undergoing therapy. The therapist, by means of vigilance and attention during the whole session, is excluded from the treatment, exercising control so as not to be affected by the colour-flooding of the therapy room. In addition, a dark blue dress or coat is a very good protection.

The treatment rhythms are based on the golden mean measurement, and are here given as measurements of time. Each number will represent a quarter of a minute. Thus $8 = 2$ minutes in time, etc. Each treatment session lasts about 35–45 minutes, including the preparation and the closing of the session. The actual colour treatment should last 24 minutes and 15 seconds.

The golden mean progression in numbers (here transposed into time) is as follows:

$1 - 2 - 3$ is too rough to use and so basic that it is seen as equal time measurement. However 3 is arrived at by the addition of $1 + 2$; thus the next – and in our case the first useful step – is 3 progressing to 5 ($2 + 3 = 5$). It becomes obvious that $3 + 5 = 8$ and we now come to the whole scale used here: $3 - 5 - 8 - 13 - 21$.

Now the treatment colour is on the increasing scale upwards, and the complementary colour on the decreasing scale downwards. Thus we arrive at:

A	=	3	5	8	13	21
B	=		21	13	8	5

A is the treatment colour
B is the complementary colour; the colours
    are alternating, A on the increase and
    B on the decreasing time rhythm

Each number in this table is divided by 4, e.g. $3 \div 4 = \frac{3}{4}$ minute or 45 seconds.

Before we look at the table which can now be followed for the treatment, we must explain the counter-movement introduced by the use of the complementary colours. It has been clearly shown from bio-feedback instruments that the effectiveness of the treatment colour is stepped up by use of the complementary colour and that the proportion introduced is vital for better results. The reduction of blood pressure, or the increase in exhaling, is very noticeable on the second and consequent 'reversal' of coloured light.

Obviously we can train a person fairly quickly to operate an existing colour therapy room and we could use electric light, but ideally we should use daylight whenever possible.

In Table 6.1 A = the treatment colour, and B = the supporting complementary colour. Times are set out in seconds, minutes and cumulative 'total' time. The room is flooded with blue before the patient enters and remains filled with this colour until treatment begins. No other light should be admitted into the room. After treatment the room is returned to the original blue until the patient has left.

TABLE 6.1   TIMETABLE FOR COLOUR TREATMENT

		Minutes	*Seconds*	*Total Time*
Start	A	0	45	0·45
	B	5	15	6·00
	A	1	15	7·15
	B	3	15	10·30
	A	2	—	12·30
	B	2	—	14·30
	A	3	15	17·45
	B	1	15	19·00
	A	5	15	24·15

Just as a doctor will not use the same words when describing an identical treatment to two different nurses whom he has got to know, so too we acquire a natural way to use the correct colour and timing for each individual. If the patient falls asleep during treatment he can be woken by gradually increasing the light to daylight level.

However, it may very often turn out that the patient does not really have a physical condition but a mental condition of asthma. Finding this to be the case, we will soon, through conversation with the patient, reach the point that he or she is able to realise that a sleep has been experienced without the usual fear of an attack of asthma. It is there that the therapist can start to help very significantly. The mental block can be removed and the patient be told that there is no reason for this asthma to continue, as the mental adjustment will remove the condition at the moment when the patient is ready to believe that asthma is not inevitable.

In a case, however, where there is a genuine asthmatic condition, we will find out in the diagnosis using the spine chart which was described earlier. If there is a reaction on dorsal 3 vertebrae, this would confirm that there is indeed a respiratory problem to be treated. There is usually also some other point or points to be considered. I have never found as yet a spine with only one point that showed a reaction; one major and two or three minor reactions will usually be found.

The vertebrae will indicate the colour and the sounds needed to be considered for the complete treatment.

EXAMPLE CASE

Asthma: *Colour Treatment*   *Shape*

Release of illness:	Blue-violet-blue	42+43
Rhythm change:	orange-yellow-orange	5

This was the psychosomatic condition. Now, having removed this, the actual findings need to be analysed. Via the doctor, the colour therapist has already discussed the suspicion of his findings and the appropriate steps have been taken to test them in any way necessary, so there is no time lost.

Arthritis:

Vertebra	Treatment Colour		Complementary Colour		Sound Intervals
C6+	Yellow I	46	Violet III	25	F–D
D2++	Magenta II	13	Green II	24	C–B
D9–	Red II	6	Turquoise II	16	C–D
L3–	Yellow III	46	Violet I	25	E–A

+ = strong impulse in diagnosis
− = weak impulse in diagnosis

It appears from the findings that here we must take the major area C6 and D2 into consideration first, as the lower D9 and L3 may be reflexes which are treated with the first couple of imbalances. If the patient needs anchoring into the physical, it is good to treat the first area and then the second. One should never treat more than one aspect in one day. It is important to treat the dominant first and clear this before moving down to the next. For a patient who is too much in the physical it can be reversed.

The numbers of these filters refer to Rank Strand Electric Ltd 'Cinemoid' (sixty-four theatrical filters which can be used when glass is not possible to obtain). It is wise to be very aware of the colours and 'ask' for their highest possible service in the name of the spirit who is called to help in the treatment. I know many doctors who, were it not for the prayers which they quietly offer to the spirit, would by now themselves be very ill. The responsibilities which are demanded of them are of a kind which are rarely, if ever, carried by any living man alone.

Massage

Not every colour therapist is a trained masseur and therefore it is important to note that the following method has been found to work in trained or untrained massage.

A masseur can work with the consciousness level merely by gently laying his hand on to the body of the patient and letting the fingers penetrate in consciousness to the place that needs the toning up by way of the mind. It is the spirit that allows the energies to go to the right place, even if it is deep inside the body. Use no force. It has happened that, in this gentle way, using the spiritually centred mind of the therapist, the mal-adjusted part has been rectified almost without the actual touch being stronger than a *gentle* push with the fingers. Also remember that a body has in its perfection a beautiful symmetry and therefore use your hands in this symmetrical way. This becomes a real 'dynamic symmetry', which was the art of the ancient Greeks who were able to work with nature and man.

Scanning

Scanning is a tried and tested method of using the heart, hands and head (mind) of the therapist to clear a patient's body.

Our hands are very sensitive organs and are used in this case as conductors of the healing energy of God. All humans have this potential and it can be trained. Great care must be taken that the process is fully understood when the training is given. The teacher must establish a good link with the student and not only a technical, intellectual one.

Scanning works directly or by proxy or even by the mental visualisation of an absent patient. Father Andrew Glazewski used to comb through a body which was not present at the moment of healing by raising the image of the person in need.

For this method to be successful we scan twice over the body of the patient, keeping in mind a colour found to be necessary at the moment; let us say blue. Blue is generally acceptable in most cases and has a general healing quality. Some of the other colours may be used as and when found to be needed at that moment. Now make a first connection with the patient from your heart, and then use both hands moving from the head to the feet of the patient, knowing that you must appeal to God within you for the healing power to flow through you.

In the first two scannings, keep your hands 3½–4½ inches away from the body. Be aware of the reactions you feel and check your findings at the end of each scanning. Finally, in the third scanning, place your hands where you have been guided to and let the energy flow through you to heal that part of the body.

CASE OF BURST APPENDIX

S.R., aged sixteen, was in hospital in September 1972. Two operations to clear the cavity of the bowels had been unsuccessful, and the patient was in a coma. It was a Thursday and nine friends had been with us, among them the patient's brother, A. The meditation group decided that they would try and help. A. offered to be proxy for his brother, we scanned S.R. (represented by A.). S.R. was reported on Friday to have woken up out of the coma, much strengthened, and on Saturday to be strong enough for a third operation which turned out to be successful.

The most outstanding observation is that all members felt positively disposed towards the experiment. It is certain that this is due to the shape we had in mind. We had all been in touch with the Pentagondodecahedron as a form of completeness to strengthen the etheric energies for our friend. The shape is also used as an instrument for treatment.

There seems an affinity of this shape with the human physical and mental structure. Colour and shape must be used in conjunction in this work of colour therapy.

The adopted shape of the colour therapy room (which is a working model of a more permanent structure, planned to be twice the size see Plate 3 (pages 84–93) is that of the last of the five Platonic regular solid bodies: the Pentagondodecahedron. Each side of each face of the working model measures 5 feet 10 inches.

The six upper faces accommodate the colour filters which these carry the six Goethian colours: blue, green, yellow, orange, red, violet. Each window, having a pentagram shape, is equipped with a fully controllable shutter. At present all experiments use daylight, which is the best light so far available to man.

Affinity to shape

The affinity of the human body with the pentagon is quite clearly visible in the human anatomy.

(*a*) The whole body can take up the position by which the extreme tips of hands and feet and the crown of the head stand in an equal-sided pentagon (Figure 6.8).

(*b*) The cross-section of the larynx has the shape of the pentagon: in the male a 90-degree and in the female 120-degree angle (Fig 6.7).

Figure 6.8   How the human anatomy fits inside a pentagon shape.

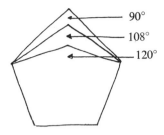

90° to 108°=interval of 18=3×6=3   3×exhaling
108° to 120°=interval of 12=2×6=2   2×inhaling

Figure 6.9   Cross-section of the larynx.

Affinity to Mentality

As mentality is intimately connected with the thinking process, this relationship now moves into the third dimension. We now have to see a solid body with twelve equal-sided pentagonal faces. Here we can find the twelve signs of the zodiac, the twelve months in the year and twice twelve hours in the day. Steiner also connects the twelve world philosophies with the human thinking activity. Hippocrates (465 BC) groups the human race into four main temperaments. There are sanguine, melancholic, choleric and phlegmatic. In the search for a meaningful connection between the shape and the temperaments, the colours associated with the latter are very deeply involved. In such a short summary it is not possible to do this subject justice as it involves a long survey of colour and its psychological meaning, as understood in our research and outlined in earlier chapters. We can only state here that each of the four temperaments is linked with a basic colour and that each of these temperaments also contains the other three. It must suffice to say that there are four groups of three pentagons which, between them, make up the whole Pentagondodecahedron. Although such knowledge is today scarcely available to the average person, sixteen volunteers responded to a colour exposure experiment in a positive way. They must all have felt subconsciously in sympathy with the shape. It was as if they were aware of this affinity.

The reader may like to go back to Chapter 3 and compare the forms and colours given there with the knowledge he has gained from the rest of the book. A person is really divided into four groupings, each grouping being composed out of three pentagons: spirit (mentality); soul, psyche (emotions); body, physical (instrument).

Thus, inside the colour therapy room, is possible to establish a harmony which has a positive reaction. We are certain that a cube of similar dimensions would bring about very different emotional reactions.

Rhythms and Colour

Although the average relative speed of breathing to pulse beat in adults is 18:72 (1:4) the colour changes take into account not only the breath and pulse rhythms, but also the mental reaction to these changes. The adjustment of the mentality takes a set period according to strength, hue and the individual person's make-up. The colour red takes a longer period than blue to slip into the subconscious perception. The time factor involved requires further investigation.

Colour used in a rhythmic change points towards an ideal form of therapy. Colour changes are capable of influencing breathing rhythms and, since every human breathes (indeed all creatures breathe, even members of the plant kingdom and mineral world), it is the basis of our well-being or otherwise. We think that very detailed research into this matter would be justified. Exposure to red results in alerting the mind, raising emotional responses and enhancing activity. These reactions are calmed and slowed down by the influence of blue light.

The four basic temperaments, as defined by Hippocrates, were the foundation on which Rudolf Steiner built. He referred to these in his educational work and also dealt with them extensively in a lecture course: 'Macrocosm and Microcosm' (Vienna, 1910).

Turn back to page 29 and see the design of the Tetrahedron in relation to the four temperaments of man.

As stated above, the basic colours are all linked to one of the temperaments of the human being and a complete balance would not normally be attainable. This colour coding may well shed some new light on to the character traits of a person in today's setting of the Western world.

Each of the four temperaments has within it the rudiments of the other three. Although there is a balancing-out process taking place in the course of maturation, the dominant basic colour will still play a significant part in a mature person's make-up. A closer look at the colours related to each of the basic temperaments will offer great opportunities for the better understanding of the human being.

In order for an ill person to find a remedy, most doctors have to rely on drugs of different kinds today. Some, but comparatively few, prescribe homoeopathic remedies. The understanding of illness today is such that most people expect relief at a faster rate than is humanly possible. They hardly ever consider that the illness itself has often developed over a long period before the point where treatment becomes necessary. A sudden restoring of the balance, by way of chemicals, is likely to be a much cruder process than the very gradual accumulation of the wrong chemical constellations or formulae which have caused the illness. Hence it becomes unavoidable, when using allopathic medicaments, for a counter-drug to be administered because the first has caused the balance to be thrown too far the other way.

This, of course, is only a very simplified pronouncement, which no doubt has far finer and more complicated implications. Here it is only intended to illustrate the point that, whilst it is necessary to use drugs in some cases, in others it would be far better to cure more slowly so as to allow the mind of the treated person to adjust to, and indeed to contribute in, the restoration of the balance in health. Therefore, a homoeopathic remedy can serve a far more harmonising purpose than a short-term allopathic drug when considering the whole of the human being.

This departure from the main theme of this summary was necessary in order to stress the point that it is really a question of how *little* need be used to restore a balanced, healthy constellation. In colour therapy we deal with very fine forms of 'medicaments', e.g. coloured lights can change such minute, though important, parts of the human chemical constellation that, if they are in the light of careful research, we will ultimately find that this therapy is capable of replacing some of the drugs which are used today.

Conclusion

Research must go hand in hand with our treatment, which we hope to begin as soon as possible. It is obvious, in the light of what has been said, that animals are not suitable subjects for our research, quite apart from the fact that we do not feel justified in using these defenceless creatures. Man can adjust his mind to conditions which cause distress in animals, by way of the mental persuasion that this is not bad or dangerous, likely to cause illness, etc., and also by sheer conscious will-power which man can strengthen according to his education and character).

Anchoring Density after Healing

When healing has been given – whether the patient is present or absent – it is important that the healer (the person through whom this healing flows) takes care to anchor the densities which he has drawn out of the aura, etheric and physical. Before even these three are being helped by the healer, the contact and prayer the healing has touched, or should have touched, the divine and the personality of the patient.

Rudolf Steiner calls the fourth ego (the divine), spirit-self. These terms refer to aspects of the whole being of man. It becomes quite clear, then, that the visible part of man is minute compared with the invisible etheric, aura, etc.

Divine (spirit-self)	=	Ether
Personality (ego)	=	Fire
Astral soul	=	Air
Etheric body	=	Water
Physical body	=	Earth

In this order appears the density or incarnation level of all visible living matter by which we are surrounded on this planet.

After a healing has taken place, the final 'ceremony' is as follows. The healer touches earth, a table, a wall or the floor. At the touch he will offer the density to the mineral kingdom and ask the state of that part of the patient's body which has

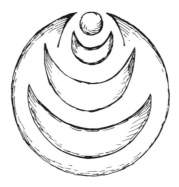

Figure 6.10   The human being as a symphony of the five elements, or

The being, (according to Rudolf Steiner) of

Physical Body	Life Body
(Earth)	(Water)
Astral Body	Ego
(Air)	(Fire)

Spirit
(Ether)

received treatment. In my experience I become aware of a figure 8 in a three-dimensional way (like two balloons). In a healthy person, or when a good balance has been achieved through the healing, the image that appears is about ⅕ above and ⅘ below where I have my hand placed. The upper half of the 8 is magenta and the lower part is green.

This indicates that the present state of the exchange in the patient is good. Any variant of this will naturally indicate an imbalance. It also suggests that the replacement tissue ratio is good.

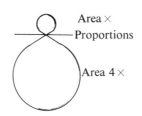

Area ×
Proportions
Area 4 ×

Where this is not balanced too much of the density has been retained by the patient and there is cause for concern.

Next we immerse our hands in water and ask how the state in this realm is. We are now in the fluid element. Here we have the etheric body which in a healthy person will look something like this:

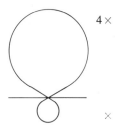

⅘ above and ⅕ below the point of touch. The upper part appears blue and the lower part orange. (This varies between individuals; bear in mind that we are each working out our own healing method.) Again, if too much of the water element is exchanged there is a draining of energy in that body. In other words, the etheric energy is being 'watered down'.

Now we come to the astral (aural). This should be very much like a pear shape but upside down – a version of the curves of Cassini. Here we have to do with the personality of the individual; and with momentary, temporary and (comparatively speaking) permanent colours, forms and balances.

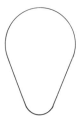

In all this is expressed so much of the personality, the soul: contentment, fear, love, hate, sadness, joy. No two auras are the same; and no aura remains static for any length of time. However, like the individuality, amazing changes take place continually, one balancing the other. Problems are invited and immediately met with the necessary energy to cope, unless we are blocking ourselves (at which we are past masters); no other being on this planet blocks so efficiently his/her own path as man.

The fourth state, air, is the ego, the personality of the patient and we are concerned with a ray body – it should be like a many-pointed star (three-dimensionally raying out in all directions). If some of the rays are weak or badly used (blocked), then this star appears very uneven or distorted. Yellow and violet mix in a luminous way, the yellow tending towards gold.

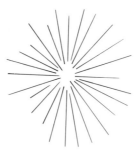

Lastly we have the etheric energy which is not to be confused with the etheric body of the individual person. This appears in a perfect circle, or rather in a beautiful sphere lit with brilliant white, but not dazzling; there are gold specks, and some very fine, exquisite green lines – so fine and clear that ordinary words cannot describe this. The orb appears to be centred where my hand is touching – centred itself and penetrating the whole field. This can be dim – or 'not able to shine through' is a better expression.

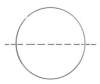

From all this (see Figure 6.9) the 'healer' can 'read' the stage which the patient has reached, or is working towards. For this to become mature and helpful, much practice is needed: not for its own sake, but because of the need to become sufficiently skilled to take up the challenge to ask for healing flow through you. Even the novice can heal; the level he/she is reaching can at times be very significant because there is no complex terminology, technique – call it what you will – in the way.

It is, however, foolish to assume that no training should therefore be given. We all have to work through the depth of consciousness and come out the other side, knowing and trusting the cause.

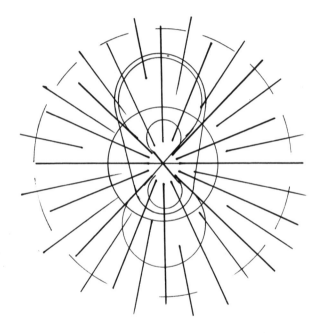

Figure 6.11   The five images which the healer should become aware of to check the health pattern of his patient, superimposed.

Coloured Light and Health: a Summary

RED   Of all the colours the most powerful, red should be used most wisely and carefully. It is vitalising, stimulating, arousing; promotes inhalation; raises blood pressure. (Sacral Gland)

ORANGE   This is the colour of joy; anti-depressant, promoting good digestion, beneficial to most of the metabolic system; rejuvenating and vitalising, it can also raise blood pressure. (Adrenals)

YELLOW   This colour gives a sense of detachment, stimulating the nervous system and promoting insecurity. It can help with the treatment of arthritis by removing density deposits in the body. (Solar Plexus)

GREEN   Just like red, this colour must be used most carefully. It has, as the complementary colour to red, the opposite effect on the body, promoting the dissolving of virgin cell structure but also the inverted cells. Heart palpitations can result through the use of this light. (Cardiac Plexus)

TURQUOISE   Refreshing and cooling, turquoise is restful for the nervous system and inflammations, also helping to cure eczema. (Thyroid Gland)

BLUE   Of all the colours this the most healing, promoting exhaling and reducing blood pressure. It is the light of peace, relaxing to the whole body, regulating the harmonious development of tissue and body structure, removing headaches and migraine, and also useful in cases of asthma. (Pituitary Gland)

VIOLET   In this colour we meet two worlds, the relaxing in the blue and the stimulating in the red. It is, in a very special way, the colour of a consciousness balance: dignity and divinity, but also stability. It will raise the self-valuation and self-esteem of the person who has lost the sense of human beauty, and restore rhythm to the system. (Pineal Gland)

MAGENTA   This colour draws man into spiritual awareness. It can be used only rarely and it would be good to keep this colour for the special purposes of the transmuting from the denser realms into the spiritual field; a colour more for the mature person.

BROWN   This implies commitment, offering, dying into matter.

GREY   The opposite of brown, grey promotes non-commitment, evasion and denial, non-involvement and escape from responsibility.

BLACK   Black draws all vibrations towards, itself sucking them in; it is the colour of self-denial.

WHITE   White insulates against all intrusion, representing purity in its extreme form. Like black it is not a colour which can be endured for long by most people.

Black and white are extremes and do not actually exist, except as density in pigment colour below red which turns into black, or when the distribution of colour is so faint as to be almost non-existent (white).

It could be said that the very dense colour of the dark shades is packed so tightly that there is no space between the molecules, but as the colour changes the packing becomes looser, so that finally we have an overwhelming amount of space into which the etheric energies can flow. Hence, with the spectrum colours in the blue range we have a much greater chance to heal, as most physical illness is caused by the accumulation of density which should have been shed before the patient became ill. (See 'Exchange breathing' in *Key, Lock and Door* by Theo Gimbel, Hygeia Publications, 1976.)

Chapter 7

An Investigation into Colour Concepts in Relation to Form

The whole idea of colour therapy has grown out of research which has been conducted with children and adults, especially prisoners and patients in mental hospitals. Some of the research is still going on, but the work completed so far is outlined here as an aid to the reader.

In our search for the reactions of the human mind to environment, and specifically to colour, as both light and as pigment, and including the form element, we have, with the help of many fine people, come to the conclusions which are here recorded.

At the present time there is an increased awareness of the importance of the quality of our environment. Design awards indicate a concern for the aesthetic standards of objects previously esteemed solely for their functional properties. New methods of dyeing, tinting and printing have evolved as safe, traditional colourways and drab monochrome uniformity have given way to adventurous and outrageous combinations of pattern and colour in dress and furnishing. Modern architecture, large-windowed, light-filled rooms and manmade fabrics have provided opportunities for experiment far beyond the dictates of necessity. There is, however, a certain monotony in the angular regularity of modern buildings, and the present tendency is to soften this harshness with lushly curving and sculptured furniture, to which many materials developed through present-day technology lend themselves.

Interior decoration and colour trends are popular features in magazines and journals; and increasingly it is being realised that the colour of our surroundings is not only artistically important but also affects us physically and psychologically.

Investigations into colour preference, the effect of colour on concentration, performance, sense of physical and mental well-being, etc., have been carried out over many years and increasing evidence has been gathered concerning the therapeutic effects of certain colours in mental health, in environment for recovery from illness, and in stimulation of the minds of young children and the mentally retarded.

However, there is little information available concerning the relationship between colour and form, and the present investigation was conceived to examine such links as exist between these two concepts. Certain colours have commonly accepted attributes or associations, which may vary from one cultural and ethnic group to another but which are generally taken for granted within the group. Similarly, certain shapes or symbols

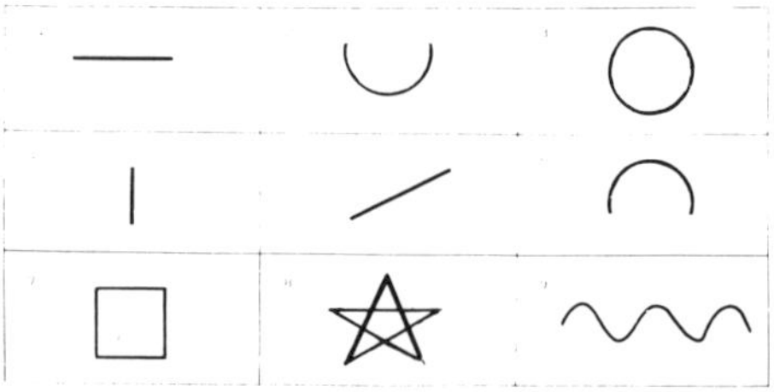

Figure 7.1   The questionnaire.

may have accepted associations or representational function within such a group; e.g. the triangle is a simple basic shape usually associated with traffic signs in Western culture.

The Shapes

Nine symbols were used in a questionnaire based on the simplest developments of the straight line and the curve (Figure 7.1).

Procedure

The questionaire used for the investigation was folded in such a way that the instructions were read before the participant saw the shapes. The instructions read:
- (*a*) Write underneath each shape the colour you think this symbol should have.
- (*b*) Take for each answer NO MORE than 10 seconds.
- (*c*) Name the shape you like like best . . . . Number . . . .
- (*d*) Name your favourite colour.

No time limit was set for the choice of favourite shape and colour. Sex and age group were recorded in the allotted space.

Analysis

More than 1,100 people completed the questionnaire and the overall trends in the group as a whole did not differ significantly from the group of 600 whose replies were analysed in detail, relating each shape to each individual colour chosen for it. The group of 600 was subdivided into 100 males and 100 females in each of the three age groups, namely, 18 years; 18–34 years; 35 years and older. The first 100 questionnaires falling into each of these six age/sex groups were used for the detailed study. They were randomly sorted. Many of the questionnaires were filled in by persons who had seen the author's letter in the *Observer* (January 1970), and had written asking for them.

Interpretation of the colours ascribed to the various shapes was necessarily simplified to twelve basic shades (see figure 7.2

and Table 7.2) so that, for example, mauve and purple were classed as violet, and scarlet, magenta and maroon were classed as red. There was no statistical significance in the differences between results obtained from each age/sex grouping so that total results have been indicated in this presentation.

Results

The colour preference indicated in question (*d*) on the research sheet is summarised in bar chart form in Figure 7.2. Blue has been the noted favourite colour for over seventy years and was named as such by 33.66 per cent of those taking part. The preference of shapes is illustrated in bar chart form in Figure 7.3. The pentagram was favoured by 34.16 per cent, followed by the circle (22.33 per cent) and the wave form (14.83 per cent). The cup shape and the square were almost equally favoured whilst the inverted cup shape and simple line forms were rarely chosen.

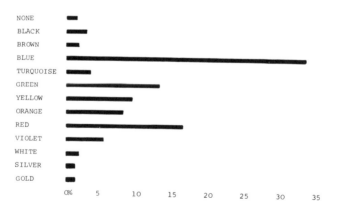

Figure 7.2   Preferred colour.

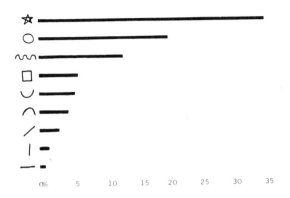

Figure 7.3   Preferred shape.

	YELLOW		BLACK		BLUE		RED .		ORANGE		GREEN	
★	233	38.83	12	2.0	67	11.13	54	11.0	22	3.83	24	4.0
O	178	29.66	16	2.66	64	10.44	176	29.33	135	22.5	29	4.83
∿	27	4.5	23	3.83	205	34.16	72	12.0	36	6.0	130	21.66
□	34	5.66	104	17.33	97	16.16	131	21.83	34	5.66	76	12.6
∪	121	20.16	15	2.5	94	15.66	103	17.16	97	16.16	76	12.6
∩	56	9.33	35	5.85	60	10.0	110	18.33	85	14.13	66	11.0
/	41	6.38	72	12.0	60	10.0	81	13.5	36	6.0	118	19.66
		26	4.33	184	30.66	57	9.5	81	13.5	15	2.5	72	12.0
—	23	3.83	226	37.66	106	17.66	71	11.83	8	1.33	65	10.83

FIG IV (cont.)

	SILVER		WHITE		BROWN		VIOLET		GOLD		TURQUOISE	
★	74	12.33	71	11.83	6	1.0	25	4.13	40	6.66	8	1.33
O	8	1.33	25	4.13	6	1.0	5	0.83	4	0.66	-	-
∿	20	3.33	13	2.18	47	7.83	35	5.85	3	0.5	24	4.0
□	14	2.33	68	11.33	41	6.83	30	5.0	3	0.5	6	1.0
∪	14	2.33	24	4.0	39	6.5	32	5.33	3	0.5	3	0.5
∩	33	5.5	25	4.13	71	11.83	56	9.33	2	0.33	6	1.0
/	44	7.33	30	5.0	60	10.0	62	10.33	-	-	8	1.33
		26	4.33	61	10.16	33	5.5	33	5.5	-	-	-	-
—	21	3.5	59	9.63	34	5.66	12	2.0	-	-	3	0.5

TABLE 7.4   SHAPE, COLOUR, NUMBER AND PERCENTAGE

The colours selected for each shape are shown in Table 7.1; 38·83 per cent of the sample chose yellow for the pentagram (shape 8) and only 2 per cent saw it as black. Conversely, the horizontal line (shape 1) was seen as black by 37·66 per cent and as yellow by only 3·83 per cent of subjects.

Discussion

In a real life situation one is not usually exposed to shapeless colour, and the limits of the colour experienced represent shape or form. The preference pattern of colour (Table 7.2) has hardly changed during the past seventy years and the present results accord with those of other workers, with blue leading in popularity (Professor Granger, May 1970, *Daily Telegraph* article.) The questionnaire did not ask for the most disliked colour, but Granger's study found it to be yellow. Modern street lighting may be yellow, white or blue. It would be of interest to note the incidence of crimes of violence committed under different lighting conditions.

TABLE 7.5   MALE/FEMALE: COLOUR, PERCENTAGE AND NUMBER

Colour	Total %	Total No.	Male %	Male No.	Female %	Female No.
BLACK	2.83	17	1.66	10	1.16	7
BROWN	2.00	12	1.16	7	0.83	5
BLUE	33.66	202	16.66	100	17.00	102
TURQUOISE	3.83	23	0.50	3	3.33	2
GREEN	12.83	77	5.33	32	7.50	45
YELLOW	9.16	55	4.66	28	4.50	27
ORANGE	8.50	51	4.16	25	4.33	26
RED	16.83	101	8.33	50	8.50	51
VIOLET	6.16	16	2.66	16	3.50	21
WHITE	1.16	7	0.50	3	0.66	4
SILVER	0.66	4	0.16	1	0.50	3
GOLD	0.66	4	0.66	4	0.00	0
NONE	1.83	11	1.33	8	0.50	3

Reactions to colour appear to be more emotional, whilst responses to shape or form seem to be more intellectual. In a classic experiment devised by *Gestalt* psychologist David Katz, small children were asked to match a green disc against an assortment of red discs and green triangles, and without hesitation they sorted the objects on the basis of colour. Adults confronted with the same task asked whether they should match for form or colour. The nine symbols used on the research sheet were simple developments from the straight line and the curve. Interpretation of these shapes was derived from information obtained from 100 volunteers aged 15–25 years, who did not take part in this project. The volunteers were asked to interpret verbally, using up to four words in 10 seconds, what the various shapes represented. The four line forms were seen as logical, physical and finite, or dead. The forms based on the curve were interpreted as illogical, spiritual and infinite, or living. The pentagram is of particular interest in that it is composed of straight lines, and yet was aligned as irregular or spiritual with the curved forms. It was seen as representative of the human form, with its five points indicating the extremities of the head and limbs, and it can be encompassed by a circle. The pentagram was the shape most favoured in the questionnaire, and was selected by 34 per cent of the sample (see Table 7.3).

TABLE 7.6   MALE/FEMALE: SHAPE, PERCENTAGE AND COLOUR

SHAPE	TOTAL %	TOTAL No.	MALE %	MALE No.	FEMALE %	FEMALE No.
——	1.00	6	0.50	3	0.50	3
∪	6.66	41	4.66	28	2.16	13
○	22.33	134	10.00	60	12.66	76
|	1.16	7	0.66	4	0.50	3
╱	4.16	25	2.00	12	2.16	13
∩	3.66	22	2.00	12	1.66	10
▢	8.83	53	6.16	37	5.50	33
☆	34.16	205	14.66	88	19.50	117
∿∿	14.83	89	8.16	49	10.66	64

The relationship of colour to form is complex and appears to be related to the interpretation of the symbols; e.g. shape no. 5 was interpreted as slope/hill/grassy/green by some individuals filling in the questionnaire. Green was, in fact, the most favoured colour for this symbol (19·66 per cent). The choice of favourite shape was not evidently influenced by the colour allotted to it. Thus yellow ranked low in colour preference, but shape 8, the pentagram, ranked first in shape preference and was thought of as yellow by 38·83 per cent of the participants with an overwhelming lead over the other colours. The wave form, shape 9, was seen predominantly as blue (34·16 per cent) but ranked third in shape preference. Figure 7.3 illustrates the preference for curved shapes over line shapes. The square, the most favoured line shape, was seen as red by 21·83 per cent with 17·33 per cent black and 16·16 per cent blue. The square was interpreted as representing strength, logic and reassurance.

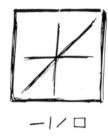

Figure 7.7   Predominant black: order of choice.

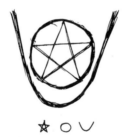

Figure 7.8   Predominant yellow: order of choice.

From Table 7.4 it may be seen that those forms seen predominantly as black are Nos 1, 4, 5 and 7, in that order of choice (Figure 7.4). Yellow predominates as the colour for shapes 8, 3 and 2 (Figure 7.4). One may conclude that little is known of the links between colour and form and their relationship to the environment in which our visual concepts have been developed. Certain ethological experiments have shown that response to form is a complex entity. Rural Zulus in South Africa know only curves in their culture; the straight line is an urban concept. Urbanised Zulus respond to the illusion, as do Europeans, whereas rural Zulus see no illusion, but are aware that the lines are of equal length. Similarly the gape reflex in young birds awaiting their feed can be elicited by displaying cardboard shapes. Research in human concepts and awareness levels are to be seen as extensions of form and size and are linked to education by which sometimes blocks occur which have to be removed when further exploration is sought.

Appendix I

Growing Plants Under Colour

The rate at which we have expanded our knowledge over the last hundred years is quite unequalled in history. Not only do we probe into the psyche of people today, but also into the reflexes of animals. More recently, research into plants has been made with the most astounding results. Peter Tompkins and Christopher Bird have made an astonishing investigation of *The Secret Life of Plants*, (Harper & Row, New York, San Francisco, London 1973). In the book *Small is Beautiful* Dr E. F. Schumacher demonstrates how plants tended by too few people produce less fruit, and how they respond to what he calls the TLC factor (tender love and care). After reading this book and exploring how plants respond to music, it seems quite natural and logical to investigate how plants respond to colour.

A few experiments were conducted to establish which type of seed would give a reasonably rapid, yet even growth rate. Of the seeds tested it was found that cress conformed admirably to these requirements. The testing and subsequent experiments were conducted scientifically, in the sense that seed was accurately weighed, the seed boxes were made to the same dimensions, etc. What to some may seem unscientific is the fact that these seeds were all treated in like fashion, not only in terms of TLC but also in physical conditions.

Procedure

On 9 August 1974 the seeds were planted in four boxes containing equal quantities of soil taken from a particular spot in a garden. The boxes were watered with an initial, carefully measured quantity, and were placed against an SSE-facing wall. Each of the boxes was individually covered with one colour filter of cinemoid, of the following numbers, from Rank Strand's selection of sixty-four colours.

Box A	=	red No. 6	primary red
Box B	=	green No. 39	primary green
Box C	=	clear No. 30	clear
Box D	=	blue No. 20	primary blue

An equal amount of air was permitted to flow into the boxes and this ventilation was arranged to exclude extra light. The seed boxes were made of wood and measured 14×8½ inches. The growing medium was 8½lb of soil at the correct moisture level for seed planting on day 1.

The results of this thirty-two-day experiment are summarised in Table A.I.1. The overall picture which emerged, however, was that within the first week red outstripped all other colours, including clear, but blue was retarded. The predicted result for green did not show until the last twelve days when, as in previous tests, the plants practically disappeared; whereas under blue they outgrew all the other boxes in length, size and development, and the taste was distinctly better, even when compared with the clear box. See Table A.I.2.

We think there must be a really remarkable change in the whole growth pattern throughout the development which depends on the colour filters. The change must be a chemical one, which ultimately caused the plants under green light to disintegrate. Between 21 August (day 13) and 9 September (day 32), the red box had grown into small and over-long seedlings, without further developing full foliage. The green, although developing more foliage, started to diminish fairly rapidly between day 18 and day 21, until on day 28 there was very little growth left. The growth in the clear box showed normal development. From day 21 under the blue filter the plants developed offshoots and spread all round in very nice order of growth. We had not allowed for 5½ inches height and so the seedlings began to touch the filter and had to bend over in order to expand.

Results

On 9 September (day 32), J. Watson, K. Loynes and myself checked together the boxes and found the results set out in Table A.I.1.

Discussion

The plant is a very useful being when taken as a measurement for later transfer to humans. Its root system can be related to man's nervous system, the foliage to the respiratory system and the flowers to the metabolic (reproductive) system. Through the insight gained from many other research projects, we believe that we can draw some parallels for discussion. For example, there is a possibility of offering this light (colour) treatment as an auxiliary means of help in cases where growth of the malignant type is found in human beings.

TABLE A.1.1
RESULTS OF GROWING SEEDS IN DAYLIGHT UNDER COLOURED FILTERS

Red   Growth: even but stunted and small foliage, almost no offshoots from stems of plants $2\frac{1}{2}$ inches high.
       Colour: light green to white stems
       Texture: elastic and could be stretched to $\frac{1}{4}$ inch before breaking
       Taste: very bitter, unpleasant to eat

Green   Growth: only fourteen very weak plants were left (see plates), 2 inches high, no offshoots
       Colour: almost white, a little faded green
       Texture: very brittle
       Taste: sharp, but no real taste

Clear   Growth: well-developed with offshoots from stems of plants $3\frac{1}{2}$ inches high
       Colour: strong, even green
       Texture: strong (normal); $\frac{1}{8}$ inch elasticity before breaking
       Taste: sweet, sharp (normal)

Blue   Growth: very well developed; up to four offshoots on each plant; largest leaf; all varieties of foliage from tiny first leaves to final top leaves; very regular in development; $5\frac{1}{2}$ inches high
       Colour: a clear strong green
       Texture: strong (normal); $\frac{1}{8}$ inch elasticity before breaking
       Taste: sweet, sharp, enhanced flavour of plant very acceptable to eat

Condition of Soil on Day 32
     Red   –   damp
     Green   –   very damp, almost sludgy
     Clear   –   a little damp (say, just right)
     Blue   –   dryish, but good moidture content for growth

TABLE A.1.2 GROWTH CHART

Over 32 days—9 August to 9 September 1974

Day	Temperature		Weather	Water	Growth / Notes				Germination %			
					R	G	C	B	Red R	Green G	Clear C	Blue B
1	15°C	10 a.m.	——	1 pt. per box	¼ oz. sown in each box				0	0	0	0
4	13°C	10 a.m.	///	1 pt. per box	Seedlings just showing				50	80	5	8
5	15°C	10 a.m.	——	none	Growth just starting				65	85	15	25
6	16°C	10 a.m.	——	none	Growth just starting				85	95	35	40
7	16°C	10 a.m.	W	1 pt. per box	½ inch growth, even in all four boxes				98	98	45	50
8	16°C	10 a.m.	W	none	$\frac{1}{3}$	$\frac{1}{3}$	$\frac{1}{4}$	$\frac{1}{4}$	98	98	45	50
11	15°C	10 a.m.	W	1 pt. per box	$\frac{1}{2}$	$\frac{3}{4}$	$\frac{1}{2}$	$\frac{1}{4}$	98	98	50	55
12	16°C	10 a.m.	W	none	$\frac{3}{4}$	$\frac{3}{4}$	$\frac{3}{4}$	$\frac{1}{3}$	98	98	50	55
13	15°C	10 a.m.	——	1 pt. per box	1	1	1	$\frac{3}{4}$	98	98	50	55
18			W	none	$1\frac{1}{2}$	$1\frac{1}{4}$	$1\frac{1}{2}$	$1\frac{1}{4}$				
26			W	none	$1\frac{3}{4}$	2	$1\frac{3}{4}$	$1\frac{3}{4}$				
29			WW	1 pt. per box	2	2	$2\frac{1}{2}$	$2\frac{1}{2}$				
32			W	none	$2\frac{1}{2}$	2	$3\frac{1}{2}$	$5\frac{1}{2}$				

KEY: C = Centigrade   —— overcast   /// rain   WW clouds with sunny intervals   W sunny

Appendix II

The Human Aura

The events which precede physical manifestation of the human form are awe-inspiring. Even before the sperm of one half (what we call the being of man) fertilises the ovum of the other half, there are energy exchanges which are caused by a third being, that being who needs to come into contact with the earth. It is as if the two parents are drawn together by a spiritual magnetic energy to meet and to remember (i.e. reorder and bring to a whole) what is seemingly dispersed amongst the stars.

Thus both are immersed in the same field of forces which overshadow their souls. At the moment when their love is consummated and conception is taking place, the second stage of the aura begins. Now some more tangible energies are being called together; there appears a shift in the directional gravitation of the aura towards the woman and away from the man. It is from that moment onwards that the bond between the two parents needs today more than just a living together. He, the man, cannot follow the subsequent events and therefore it is up to the woman to communicate them to him. Through questioning he can draw out of her, the becoming-mother, knowledge which appears to have been brought to her by the soul which has started the actual manifestation process. There is no hard logic about this kind of communication; there should be a telling of a tale which requires no intellectual structuring. And it is perhaps in the pictures which are presented before the souls of both parents that much is revealed. When later, much later, the child develops into maturity before the eyes of the parents, there may then be seen more clearly why certain images during pregnancy were appearing. Most women live through these on an unconscious level, or in a dream-like way. Only when the becoming-father, in the quietness of the night, from time to time puts loving questions, can she respond by describing the images.

In this way, and only in this way, the father can support and participate in the child's development and experiences. But the mother who is privileged to have a child fathered by a man who can participate in this way will also be blessed with deeper enrichment of the soul through this process of manifestation.

What happens now to the mother who has chosen to offer the 'inner universe' in which a child can grow? There is interplay within her between the energies of balance – some which release, others which also draw together. It is as if the mind and soul of the mother reaches out into the vast expanse of the universe. And by this change which takes place within her own mind (incurred by the spiritual events which powerfully draw up the physical energies) she is 'reaching' into the cosmic consciousness and partaking in the down-flowing of the future individuality.

Two very distinct networks are being created, one by co-operation between the pineal and pituitary glands, and the other by co-operation between the thyroid gland and cardiac plexus (heart). The first is building up the whole of the nervous system, as if it were filling out the 'blueprint' of the etheric energies, already planned long before; Rudolf Steiner uses the nice image of a glove into which the hand slips. On the other side we find the throat-sound energy vibrating much more slowly and building the blood system in co-operation with the heart. Here, too, the plans are already in hand; the building takes place in accordance with these. Bear in mind that alterations will be made along the path, for reasons to be explained later in this appendix.

The complexity of the brain and the whole of the nervous systems (as there are two complementary ones in our bodies) stretches out in a vast network to communicate to the whole of that body. This seems to have mainly the energy of the white colour – maybe a very fine peach blossom (magenta) colour. On the psychic level the colour is brilliant but not dazzling.

The other systems (again two) are the bloodstream which is centred in the heart. Here we find the colour red, and red is the densest colour in the spectrum, while the brilliant 'white' is possibly the clearest colour. On the psychic level we see the heart as green, which is the colour of physical manifestation.

The complexity of the brain and the comparative simplicity of the heart are again a wonder; and it occurs to the seeker after truth that there are energy shifts which bring about the gradual changes that produce such metamorphoses and indicate that a complex organ – the brain – becomes an apparently much less complex but more mature organ like the heart. She has, in a way, gone 'out' to meet this soul on the cosmic level. However, this deeply subconscious (or dream-like) state of the mother accounts for the fact that many becoming-mothers, during the 280-odd days of pregnancy, often have new ideas, altered styles of living, desires to eat other foods; in short, they are in a changing world.

The flow of the mother's soul is outward, away from her being towards that soul which draws closer and closer as the magnetic energies are filling out the form of the body, the instrument which we can only see after birth.

The mother's vacating of her own consciousness, her mind and her feeling supports the future child's energies, which are drawn down into her and set up the counterflow. She creates a vacuum which allows the new being to call into her space the soul who brings down a teaching of which modern mothers, both parents even, ought to know more. The other flow of energy is that from the realms of the material earth; the finest qualities and quantities of chemical and mineral substances are drawn up to make manifest the body.

The organisational energies are interweaving the whole time and are of two main types: (*a*) the etheric energy which is much more closely linked with the ordering of the molecular structures inside the body and the immediate vicinity of this body, and (*b*) the much larger field of the aura. The beginning of the weaving and creating process is just an interchange and exchange of matter–spirit, flow and static; in other words like a see-saw, continually exchanging images and experiences. The personality of the future child is dipping into the ordering of the etheric molecular field where this soul sets out the plan and lays down the potentials which are needed 'this time round'. The parents are really the participating onlookers and supporters of this cosmic event.

There is built now, behind the scenes as it were, a divine, perfect, beautiful aura with all its energies that exchange in and out, density and spirituality, liquid and solid. As the end of the 280 days draws near, we find that the individual is choosing to draw in what we call weaknesses, flaws, imperfections; and the aura, as well as the etheric sheath, is laying out a map of the imperfections so that this individuality can learn about perfection.

The flaws are, as it were, missing or unclear 'threads', imperfect areas and left-out energies which can then be filled with the images that the individual, later in life, will consciously select for himself. All these 'weaknesses', which we usually call disease, are doors through which the real personality can speak, supported by the spiritual energies that flow through the 'gates' which have been left uncompleted. This is where we, as individuals, can become creative.

Looking at history, it is often the weaknesses which prompt an individual to contribute new discoveries to the field of human knowledge. Potentially these are all present already, but only consciousness can really help to make out of the 'dreamer' a being who will take up the challenges which lead him to become one of the co-creators of our world(s).

As we are dealing with a physical and spiritual event, we can only see how the physical appearances are the results of the spiritual interventions. The 'master builder' is beyond the pineal and pituitary, in other words the Spirit, the God-being, who works through the glands into matter. So we can see how the pineal gland becomes the centre of the finest web in the nervous system which penetrates the body; from there the pituitary gland receives its orders to conduct the building of the body within the uterus, which is a replica of the universe. At the end of the 'master builder's' task, when at birth the child gradually begins to inhabit this temple of energies – of which part is visible to all and part visible only to a few (as yet) – he, the master-builder, seems to withdraw. The function of the pineal gland seems to be completed. Only much later, at the end of what we call puberty, does an amazing event take place; the body, now fully anchored in the earth, receives a call to find a way to that same field whence came the initial impulse to bring together the two parents. Today we are receiving a very clear appeal to remember that source; we are seeking a path back to the initial place, this time very consciously.

At about the fourteenth year of a person's life, the 'master builder' seems to start becoming active again. But the task for him now is gradually to lead the incarnated being to the place where the original energies came from. This is really a reversal of the initial task of the pineal gland. Meditation makes use of this gland and starts to imbue it with energies which were originally in the womb flowing in the other direction. Thus we can say that the whole incarnating process of an individual changes over into an excarnating one.

During a child's development we know that, step by step, a reversal of images and sounds and gravity takes place. The baby cannot stand upright until the images of sight are reversed; in other words a baby, until that moment, sees the world upside down. The same thing happens with sounds in the child. A complete reversal of sounds is necessary before the child can develop speech. Later still, the world of colour is reversed. From those crude and very general developmental stages we can now see how this principle of changeover is an on-going process. Indeed, if we were to say 'Now I am ready, I am at the goal, at the final point', there would be no reason for us to exist at all.

As soon as we have arrived in one place we must start to tackle the next step. It seems that what was once an outer task becomes an inner task; what once created matter now creates spirit – and the changing order of energies is basically the absolute law of existence.

From this we may finally deduce that all glands of the body fulfil a double task, and that not only is a one-way change made, but a total, three-dimensional evolution – revolving, exchanging, weaving of all energies – is taking place. Two parallel energies are playing the rotation game of exchange. The moment a state of equilibrium is reached, a new principle must come into play. The study of geometry is vital to our own concept of the forming and lifting of the consciousness. If we are foolish enough to hope that we can say 'It is done' and think this is the END, then indeed we must be blind. Such a concept has brought about many maladies.

When the breasts have nursed and the uterus has been a 'universe' to create a child (or maybe more than one) the mothers, by and large, find at the end that these organs are obsolete, and often neglect what were once the most important glands in their system. The nursing or pregnant mother is indeed a goddess who creates a new universe – magically, out of the invisible world, a being is growing into the visible world. The energies of both womb and breasts are involved in the flow of creation. After or during the menopause in both women and men, something takes place which is little understood and hardly known.

The grandmother who holds a baby on her lap could, if she had the knowledge, give to the child an energy which the mother as yet cannot offer. In the past these energies were changed over in the subconscious and happened very naturally. There was a feeling between mother and daughter: the daughter, who is now mother, handing her baby to *her* mother, subconsciously felt a difference in this holding. If, in the light of the above, we can see that the changes are now in need of being made by support of our own conscious concepts about them, then we can start to see how we are gradually mastering the task of the 'master builder'.

During the menopause a woman or man should consider the renewal of energies such as will enable the sexual organs to be imbued with new tasks, so that a new purpose is seen in the mature woman's breasts and her uterus. From there can now flow spiritual energies to the little receptive child, which are not those of the still-young mother.

Through meditation, the use of the pineal gland opens the gate to the spiritual return of the individual; then gradually all the ductless glands receive the new task – ending right down at the base of the spine, with what then becomes the spiritualised, enlightened centre of man, right down to the sacral gland. An inner, beautiful light becomes established and one wonders if hysterectomies and breast operations could become unnecessary if a molecular change were made through the agency of the human consciousness to allow the new flow of energy to go through these 'new organs', now fulfilling a new task, thereby re-enlivening them for a new purpose. If this is not also a logical event – i.e. the flow of metamorphosing food into heat, coal into light and all the other thousand ways in which we reverse the energies – it is also the most awe-inspiring experience that we can be aware of: the new body in a new being which evermore evolves to transmute the energies, ebbing and flowing, in and out, once visible and once invisible.

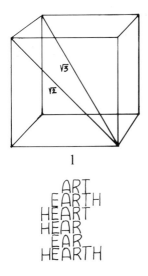

1

```
  ART
 EARTH
HEART
HEAR
 EAR
HEARTH
```

'She' and 'he' as separate beings create the complete being. This, of course, never materialises fully in the visible world.

'He' is the content energy (Figure A.II.1 that shows the star nature of most accurate energy-flows, which obey very precise laws. Content energy based on the three measurements of the temple of the new Jerusalem. In mathematical terms, this is the measure of one to root two and root three we have created the basic needs to build the measures that make the hexahedron. This, of all energies, represents earth and also the heart.

HEART
EARTH
HEARTH (the source of energy, the central place)

The second co-operating and completing energies are also the container energies for the content. This the woman, the 'she' who is the protecting and enclosing energy, however closely related to the design of 'him'.

We can see so beautifully the encircling energies, back to the womb, back to the eternal being of the two making the third. The third is invisible.

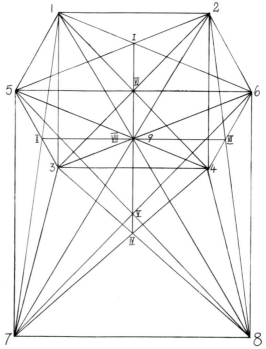

Figure A.II.1   The energy of the content.

Key: 1 – 2 – 3 – 4   Back of Hexahedron
       5 – 6 – 7 – 8   Front of Hexahedron
linked points by diagonals create a 9th point. This becomes the hermetic cross or on the two dimensional level, the Maltese cross. Linking all diagonal crossings we come from:

   II – III = horizontal
   I – IV = vertical
   VI – V = depth known as the three dimensions. This cross is known as the Christ Cross and creates a seventh VII point.

This adds up to known energy experiences in Leadbeaters work.*[1]

*The Rt. Reverend C. W. Leadbeater, *The Science of the Sacraments*. The Theosophical Publishing House, Adyr, Madras, India, 1949.

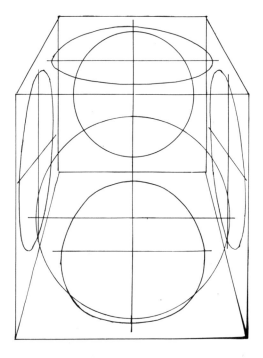

Figure A.II.2   The Energy of the Container.

The Energy of the Container

Protecting all six sides this form provides the vessel in which can securely grow the consciousness, the content. It is used in ritual work as a protection for space, a church, a sanctuary, a healing area, etc. The vessel is not mathematically determined and offers thereby a complementary energy to the content. The content can be seen as the 'male', whereas the container as the 'female' energies. A divine co-operation between the two is also a health picture for each human being. The man who holds the hidden woman invisibly within and the woman who holds the hidden man within her being. No wonder the two find each other on many levels, as the case may need, or social work or ritual actions require.

References and Further Reading

Books

Billmeyer, F. W., and Saltzman, M., *Principles of Colour Technology* (Wiley, Interscience).

Birren, F., *History of Colour in Painting* (Reinhold).

Bragg, Sir W., *The Universe of Light* (Bell).

British Colour Council, *Dictionary of Colour Standards*.

Burnham, R. W., Hanes, R. M., and Bartleson, C. J., *Colour* (Wiley).

Chevreuil, M. E., *Principles of Harmony and Control of Colours* (Reinhold).

Clifford, D., *Art and Understanding* (Evelyn, Adams & Mackay).

Cott, H. B., *Adaptive Colorative in Animals* (Methuen).

Dartnall, H. J. A., *Visual Pigments* (Methuen).

Dorfman, B., *Colour Mixing* (Pitman).

Evans, R. M., *Introduction to Colour* (Wiley).

Fletcher, G. S., *Sketching in Colour* (Allen & Unwin).

Friedman, J. S., *History of Colour Photography* (Focal Press).

Gluck, F., *World Graphic Design* (Studio Vista).

Green, A. E. S., *The Middle Ultraviolet* (Wiley).

Goethe, J. W. von, *Theory of Colour.*

Gregory, R. L., *Eye and Brain* (Weidenfeld & Nicolson).

Heard, H. G., *Laser Parameter Measurements Handbook* (Wiley).

Heel, A. C. S. van, *What is Light* (World University Library).

Hingston, R. W. G., *Meaning of Animal Colour and Adornment* (Arnold).

Homer, W. I., *Seurat and the Science of Painting* (MIT Press).

Horticultural Colour Chart (Wilson Colour Ltd).

Hunt, R. W. G., *The Reproduction of Colour* (Fountain Press).

Hutchinson, H. F., *The Poster* (Studio Vista).

Itten, J., *Art of Colour* (Reinhold).

Jaffe, B., *Michelson and the Speed of Light* (Heinemann).

Judd, D. B., and Wyszecki, G., *Colour in Business, Science and Industry* (Wiley).

Judson, J. A. V., *Handbook of Colour* (Dryad).

Kornerup, A., and Wanscher, J. H., *Methuen Handbook of Colour* (London, Methuen).

Le Grand, Y., *Light, Colour and Vision* (Chapman & Hall).

McMullen, R., *World of Marc Chagall* (Aldus).

Matthens, S. K., *Photography in Archaeology and Art* (John Baker).

Mueller, C. G., *Light and Vision* (Life Science Library).

Mueller, R. E., *The Science of Art* (Rapp & Whiting).

Neal, C. Dr, *Light and Colour* (Odhams).

Oeri, G., *Man and his Images* (Studio Vista).

Papoulis, A., *Systems and Transforms with Applications in Optics* (McGraw-Hill).

Penrose Annual 1968 (Lund Humphries).

Penrose Annual 1976 (Lund Humphries).

Popper, F., *Origins and Development of Kinetic Art* (Studio Vista).

Rao, C. N. R., *Ultraviolet and Visible Spectroscopy* (Butterworth).

Rendell, J., *Matchbox Labels* (David & Charles).

Stanley, R. C., *Light and Sound for Engineers* (Nelson).

Steiner, R., *Colour Course* (Anthroposophical Press).

Taylor, A., *Making the Most of Colour in the Home* (Arco).

Taylor, F. A., *Colour Technology* (Oxford University Press).

Voitkevich, A. A., *The Feathers and Plumage of Birds* (Sidgwick & Jackson).

Wilson, J., *Decoration U.S.A.* (Macmillan).

Wright, W. D., *The Measurement of Colour* (Hilger & Watts).

Wright, W. D., *The Rays Are Not Coloured* (Hilger & Watts).

Wyszecki, G., and Stiles, W. S., *Colour Science* (Wiley).

Journal Articles

Savidge, R., 'Colour to tame a monster', *RIBA Journal* (August 1965).

'Green light for infrared', *Nature* (18 January 1969).

Miller, H. B., '"Is red" and "Looks red"', *Mind* (July 1967).

'Light: special colour edition', *Scientific American* (September 1968).